ABORIGINAL HEALTHWORKERS

DATE DUE

ABORIGINAL
HEALTHWORKERS

PRIMARY HEALTH CARE AT THE MARGINS

BILL GENAT
with
Sharon Bushby, May McGuire, Eileen Taylor,
Yvette Walley, Thelma Weston

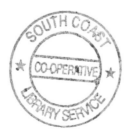

University of Western Australia Press

First published in 2006 by
University of Western Australia Press
Crawley, Western Australia 6009
www.uwapress.uwa.edu.au

Publication of this book was made possible with funding from Onmenda VicHealth
Koori Health Unit, University of Melbourne

National Library of Australia
Cataloguing-in-Publication entry:

Genat, Bill.
    Aboriginal healthworkers: primary health care at the margins.

    Bibliography.
    Includes index.
    ISBN 1 920694 76 5.
    ISBN 978 1920694 76 0.

    1. Aboriginal Australians—Medical care. 2. Aboriginal Australians—
    Services for. 3. Health services accessibility—Australia.
    4. Transcultural medical care—Australia. I. Title.

362.10899915

Consultant editor: Jean Dunn, Melbourne
Designed and typeset by Pages in Action, Melbourne
Typeset in 10.5/13pt Adobe Garamond
Printed by BPA Print Group, Melbourne

Foreword

Today, few would argue that Aboriginal and Torres Strait people experience a completely unacceptable level of health and social disadvantage. All Australian governments have agreed to strategies to improve Indigenous health—including building the capacity of the health system to respond better to needs.[1] High priority has been given to developing the capacity of the health workforce, particularly the component with a specific focus on Aboriginal and Torres Strait people. Aboriginal healthworkers have for nearly four decades played a pivotal role in the delivery of Indigenous-specific services. Accordingly, the Australian health ministers agreed in 2002 that 'improving the clarity of roles, regulation and recognition ... vocational education and training sector support' for Aboriginal healthworkers was a key objective in their workforce development strategy.[2]

A number of factors have raised the profile of Aboriginal and Torres Strait Islander health: the activism of Indigenous Australians (and the political and institutional responses); reporting and media commentary, and academic publishing. Academic commentary, like the broader public debate in which it is situated, has tended to focus on description and analysis of the health problem. With some notable exceptions, the response of Indigenous Australians to their health problems has not been well documented. The Aboriginal writer Kevin Gilbert, in his 1973 book, *Because a White Man'll Never Do It*, notably captured the political mood of a generation of Aboriginal activists who insisted that Aboriginal Australians needed to take control of their own affairs. Aboriginal communities had, from 1971, begun to establish community-controlled health services, which have grown over the years from small voluntary clinics to complex primary health care organisations.

Aboriginal healthworkers were pivotal to this new terrain. As primary care workers, they were employed by the growing number of Aboriginal community-controlled and government-run services being established across the country. They were variously described in those early days as barefoot doctors or culture-brokers, descriptions that only partially capture the complexity and diversity of their role. To some extent this role varies according to the health profile and priorities of the local community in which they work. Increasingly, healthworkers have adopted more specialist roles, such as in women's health, mental health or aged care. Although Aboriginal and Torres Strait people can be found working in nearly all health occupations, healthworkers are, after nurses, still the most common Indigenous occupational group in the health workforce (according to the 2001 census). Yet there have been very few academic studies that engage with their experiences and challenges.

Bill Genat provides rich insight into the complexity of Aboriginal healthworker practice. Attentively descriptive and highly evocative, the everyday working world of healthworkers in an urban Aboriginal community-controlled health service is brought to life. Based in the Family Care section, the healthworkers provide assistance to frail aged and disabled Aboriginal people. The experiences of healthworkers are explored, and are juxtaposed against the perspective of clients, other staff and health professionals, and community members. We get a sense of the triumphs and struggles of healthworkers, who deal both with the issues that flow from a lack of institutional and professional recognition within the broader system, and with the complex and challenging needs of their clients. The account is at times raw and revealing. Whilst it lays out many difficulties and contradictions of healthworker practice, it also documents the extraordinary commitment these workers make to their community.

This book is an important contribution to the development of Aboriginal healthworker policy and strategy. A study of this type, which gives a detailed reckoning of the lived experience and daily realities of healthworker practice, is in fact long overdue. Hopefully, it signals a growing engagement in the social sciences with workforce issues in Aboriginal health.

Professor Ian Anderson
Inaugural Chair of Indigenous Health
University of Melbourne

Contents

Tables and Figures

Abbreviations

AHS   Aboriginal Health Service
UNICEF   United Nations International Children's Emergency Fund

Preface

The health status of Aboriginal Australians continues to lag far behind that of most other Australians.[1] Indeed, recent data suggest the gap is widening.[2] While particularly evident in remote areas, this difference persists in cities and towns where, potentially, Aboriginal people have access to all available mainstream health and medical services.[3]

Aboriginal healthworkers are employed by primary health care services as a strategy to ensure that health services are not only accessible, but also culturally appropriate and acceptable to Aboriginal Australians. Nevertheless, there is much controversy about what healthworkers can and should be doing. Discontent is evident among the healthworkers themselves and among health policy-makers and clinical health professionals about healthworker practice and its substance, place and application.

This book presents a rich and detailed account of Aboriginal healthworker activities and the unique interpretations and understandings central to their work. It also reveals the interplay of diverse viewpoints within the professional context of their work. It describes the enormous complexity they face, due to historical legacies of exclusion, cultural oppression and racism that continue to erode the environmental, psychological, social and cultural health of their Aboriginal clients. Frequently, their clients are struggling with family and social problems that override personal health management and, within their own families, are enduring harmful relationships related to dependency. The healthworkers' response to the complexity of their task has been to develop a unique client-centred holistic practice. However, lack of organisational and professional recognition by managers and by more clinically oriented health professionals has compromised their efforts.

A long collaborative project between a group of Aboriginal health-workers and a researcher at an urban Aboriginal Health Service in Western Australia underpins this book. Healthworkers have generally been written about by other health professionals. Together, in a collaborative study using ethnographic methods, we sought a deeper insight into the practice of healthworkers and the meanings and understandings they bring to their work.

The origins of this study lie in a teaching programme for Aboriginal healthworkers. The group seminars with experienced healthworkers and the supervision of workplace projects revealed many of the underlying dilemmas and conflicts common amongst healthworkers. Occasional dissent between teaching staff about curriculum content highlighted a lack of systematic research and knowledge about day-to-day healthworker practice. But while these factors gave the initial impetus, it was the desire of the healthworkers to tell their own story that provided the energy and commitment necessary to complete this project. While the fieldwork was conducted in the late 1990s, the problems it identifies are little damaged.

Indigenous experience, knowledge and voices are often absent from research about Indigenous people,[4] and the intent of this book is to highlight them. As far as possible, the voices of the healthworkers precede observations and analysis of their practice by other commentators, which enables that commentary to be re-viewed through an Indigenous lens.

Numerous people inspired and assisted with the development of this project. Foremost, we acknowledge and thank the other Aboriginal healthworkers who made this study possible: Irene Bartlett, Vicki Blurton, Jocelyn Gabrielson, Janeena Humphreys, Harold Miller, Irene Nannup, Jacque Page, Marjorie Winmar and Sharryn Yarran. Likewise, we thank the two Aboriginal care-aides, Rhonda Spikes and Sharon Taylor. We would also like to thank the other employees of the Aboriginal Health Service, in particular Ted Wilkes, the Director. Dr Ernie Stringer and Dr Peter Underwood both provided supervision, support and genial hospitality throughout. Kathryn Shain provided editorial support, a warm sense of humour, patience and camaraderie. *Onemda* VicHealth Koori Health Unit at the University of Melbourne generously provided a grant that was essential to the publishing of this book. Maureen de la Harpe and her staff at UWA Press guided publication of the text, with Jean Dunn as editor. Heartfelt thanks, and may this book benefit all workers committed to the struggle for better health.

Bill Genat

At the Frontline

Ruby, in her mid-twenties, slumps gloomily at the kitchen table, brooding on the potential of healthworkers to change the status of Aboriginal health. As we drink tea, she shares her reflections with me and with Merle who, like Ruby, is an Aboriginal healthworker:

> They wanted all us healthworkers 'cause we were going to change everything, but we're so strictly dictated to, it's changed nothing. Some of us have great ideas, and we could do it all, but we just can't do it ... we don't get enough say in the programme.

The staffroom of the Family Care section of the Aboriginal Health Service (AHS) is the kitchen of an old house converted to offices. The kitchen table stands in the centre of the room. Underneath the chimney, where previously a wood-fired stove sat, rests an old metal instruments trolley with a microwave and a toaster on it. Near the doorway to a storeroom stands the fridge, and next to it a stainless-steel sink with numerous coffee mugs draining. The fridge supports a couple of fridge magnets, radio bumper stickers, and a squat, portable radio/cassette, which usually pours out 1970s easy-listening music and news reports. The radio is off, but the phones constantly ring, and clients and staff pass back and forth on their way to other offices.

Merle recounts the morning's events, including a harrowing tale of Teddy, a young, Aboriginal client disabled by complications from non-insulin-dependent diabetes. Teddy had been discharged from hospital to his home, where Merle visited him next day:

> **Merle**: I don't know what made me decide to dress his foot. I said to him, 'Before I go, I better have a look at that foot of yours'. So I unwrapped it, and it hadn't been done. He said they did it at the hospital once. It stunk, it had maggots in it—so anyway, I cleaned it up as much as I could and put a bandage on it.
>
> The toes were black, and I said, 'Are you sure that they dressed it only once?' 'No, no', he said, 'They only dressed it once'. So now he's gonna lose his toe over that. So then Ruby went up [to the District Hospital to visit him] on Friday, afternoon ...
>
> **Ruby**: Ooh man, he was in pain, crying, poor little thing. He had a fever, 39.5° ... They gave him an antibiotic straight into the vein and he looked better, but the toe it was black—it was split, oozing ... Now I understand why he doesn't like the hospital, because obviously they just neglected him there.
>
> Well, when I went to the hospital, I said, 'Look this man got discharged from hospital yesterday. A healthworker dressed his toe this morning and found maggots in it'.
>
> She said, 'He couldn't 've had maggots in it'.
>
> I said, 'He had maggots in his toe!'
>
> 'Are you sure they were maggots?'
>
> I said, 'Yes'.
>
> 'They couldn't have ...'
>
> That was at the District Hospital, and at the General Hospital they said the same thing to me.
>
> **Merle**: They didn't even believe Ruby—that he'd been just discharged the day before ... I wouldn't have noticed the maggots, only they started wriggling.
>
> **Ruby**: Ooh man, I'm glad I didn't find them. I just can't understand why they discharged him.

Teddy's story is one example of the practice of Aboriginal health-workers in the Family Care section of the Aboriginal Health Service. Much of their work is hands-on, outside the clinic, at street level and in client homes. Their clients are often in physical pain, and suffer from chronic illnesses, injury, recent surgery, side-effects of medication, not taking their medication, taking incorrect dosages and confusing their medications. Their clients reflect contemporary Aboriginal urban life in Australia: a realm for many of unemployment and poverty, overcrowded rental households with constant risk of eviction and where drugs and alcohol trigger emotional and physical pain—with a history of exclusion and repression where the death of loved ones is a constant companion.

Removed from the professional and organisational structures that in a hospital or clinic separate private and public space, Aboriginal healthworkers daily face realities invisible to others. Professional distance, ignorance or both may have prompted the nurse's dismissal of Ruby's inquiries about Teddy. Ironically, the event denies the Aboriginal healthworker's unique, local professional experience—the very experience supposedly valued in the notion of community healthworker or 'barefoot doctor'.

THE POLICY CONTEXT

Three major Commonwealth government reports published since the early 1990s state that the social and environmental factors underlying the inferior health status of Indigenous Australians are the legacy of colonial oppression.[1] The Royal Commission into Aboriginal Deaths in Custody (1991) reported:

> The key determinants of the health of Aboriginal people today ... are found in the history of Aboriginal people and in their current social and physical environments ... Two centuries of oppression, combined with poverty, health damaging physical environments, social disruption and poor diets combine to produce the poor health status of Aboriginal people today.[2]

Almost ten years later, the House of Representatives Standing Committee on Family and Community Affairs identified the same factors, and emphasised the effects of alcohol misuse, high levels of tobacco consumption, distance from services and lack of cultural awareness among health personnel.[3] This report showed that three out of four Aboriginal deaths resulted from diseases of the circulatory system (heart attacks and strokes), injury and poisoning (road accidents, suicide and murder), respiratory diseases (pneumonia, asthma and emphysema), neoplasms (cancers) and endocrine, nutritional and metabolic disorders (such as diabetes).

A limitation of this type of epidemiological data is that it rarely reveals the social and cultural factors that lead to poor Aboriginal health or ineffective delivery of health services. Yet from the ealy 1970s, the importance of the social and cultural components of service delivery was recognised, and Aboriginal people were employed within Aboriginal health programmes. This strategy held great promise for more accessible and appropriate services.

ORIGINS OF HEALTHWORKER PRACTICE

Indigenous healthworker practice has a long history. In the 1920s colonial administrations employed Primary Health Workers (PHWs) across Asia and Africa to dispense Western healing concepts and practices across the cultural divide. Walt reports that until the early 1980s, PHWs worked as druggists, disease-specific treatment providers, first-aiders, vaccinators and health promoters.[4] Revelations of the central role of the barefoot doctor in China as a provider and mobiliser of health care gave added impetus,[5] and the landmark Alma Ata Declaration on Primary Health Care, with its vision of 'Health for All' further formalised and promoted the concept of PHWs.[6]

According to Walt, UNICEF and the World Health Organization (WHO) envisioned PHW programmes as pivotal to the implementation of the Alma Ata Declaration, and particularly to the emphasis on cultural appropriateness, community participation and self-determination.[7] The WHO proposed that PHWs should be selected and supported by their own community, provide a link to the community, relieve professionals of routine treatments, provide both preventative and curative services, mobilise community action on health and be accountable to both the community and the government.[8] Importantly, the WHO envisaged that healthworkers would cost less than highly trained professionals.[9] Subsequently, many Asian, Latin American and African countries developed national PHW programmes.

This international movement stimulated the employment and training of Indigenous Australians to deliver primary health care services to Aboriginal people.[10] During the late 1960s the Health Department of Western Australia recruited a small number of Aboriginal healthworkers in the Kimberley region. In 1973 this programme received a financial boost and encouragement from the community-oriented health and welfare policies of the newly elected federal Labor government. The federal government also gave impetus to the Aboriginal Medical Services, which had been established in the early 1970s[11] and which also employed Aboriginal healthworkers.

The initial conceptions of Aboriginal healthworker practice broadly paralleled those in the international development context.[12] They emerged in optimistic reports from medical doctors within the Northern Territory health department.[13] In line with these ideas, Soong proposed a broad scope of practice for healthworkers, including basic medical care, personal health care (health education), community health action and, notably, health service management.[14] This is notable because in less developed countries PHWs were expected merely to administer rather than to manage.[15] Ultimately, Aboriginal communities resisted the policy of Aboriginal management of government health clinics in their communities,[16] and thus political expediency also played a role in shaping healthworker practice.[17]

During this early phase of development, Aboriginal healthworkers performed, in theory, most of the tasks assigned to PHWs in the international context. However, Soong gave particular emphasis to one aspect of practice: healthworkers as 'cultural brokers' to further the agendas of clinical professionals.[18] He viewed healthworkers as communication agents employed on the one hand to transmit clinical information to Aboriginal clients, and on the other to relay social and environmental data concerning clients back to the clinic. Within the

Health Department of Western Australia during the 1970s and 1980s, this broking or 'liaison' role officially defined almost all healthworker practice, although some isolated healthworkers had, out of necessity, more clinical responsibilities than their city counterparts.[19]

Aboriginal medical services were not government-run, and they fashioned healthworker practice quite differently. According to Joan Winch, they viewed healthworkers more as practitioners in their own right.[20] In addition to liaison and health education roles, their healthworkers practised as basic clinicians and advocates. Consequently, within Western Australia the roles and training of healthworkers came to differ between the government and the non-government sectors. Disparate organisational, geographic and professional contexts, each encompassing particular agendas, needs and expectations, produced a diverse array of healthworker tasks. As a result, healthworkers are identified with a wide range of practice.

Amidst these local developments, some serious limitations to PHWs' role as vanguard of a new Health for All were recognised in the international literature. Researchers found that PHW practice exhibited a curative rather than a preventive focus,[21] minimal community accountability,[22] a lack of cultural appropriateness,[23] increasing professionalisation and identification with the clinic[24] and professional jealousy about status within the health care team.[25] According to Skeet, the perceived scope of PHW practice was impossible to implement:

> Responsibility for implementation of the Alma Ata Declaration at the village level—home visits, environmental sanitation, provision of safe water supply, first aid for injuries, treatment of simple and common ailments, health education, nutritional surveillance, maternal and child health ... a list of this kind would daunt a professional health worker, surely it is absurd to expect village workers to shoulder it?[26]

Berman and colleagues, and Walt, suggested that organisational inadequacies in training, supervision and supplies incapacitated PHW practice.[27] Walt specifically emphasised how patterns of power relations in the wider society affected PHWs in the workplace. Gender and class differences in relation to other professionals and clients resulted in PHWs facing inequality and conflict.[28] Walt reported that medical professionals (predominantly male doctors) promoted healthworker programmes, but nurses were rarely consulted and remained uninformed. As a result, nurses often treated PHWs as their assistants.[29] Walt suggested that the contextual constraints on PHW practice were largely unforseen by medical professionals.

Similarly, contextual constraints on Aboriginal healthworker programmes were largely unanticipated. Willis indicated that within the Northern Territory healthworker programme, doctors controlled policy and administration.[30] They rarely consulted nurses who worked with healthworkers, and were generally ignorant of the day-to-day issues. In particular, they were unaware of tensions between healthworkers and nurses.

Incongruously, it was also reported that healthworkers faced cultural barriers in the form of lack of community co-operation, or 'resistance'. Explanations for this included the lack of status of young women employed as healthworkers;[31] the lack of status of healthworkers compared to traditional healers and to medical doctors;[32] and community conflict over employer expectations that healthworkers advocate behaviour changes to people who were their senior in kinship terms.[33] According to Folds, healthworkers confronted community resistance to 'assimilationist practices'.[34]

A comprehensive Northern Territory report in the late 1980s documented professional, cultural, educational and practical constraints on day-to-day healthworker practice.[35] It found that, in professional terms, nurses mentored healthworkers, who worked mostly as their clinical assistants. The programme was largely unsupported by other health professionals, who often lacked cultural awareness. The few preventive and educative components of healthworker practice lacked community support and were inhibited by cultural prohibitions and fears of 'payback'. The report suggested that the primary health care model of service delivery was undermined by a lack of educational role models and that healthworkers were subject to unrealistic expectations, given their training. It recorded accounts of healthworkers caught between competing community and employer demands, and found that the high clinical morbidity in Aboriginal communities meant that there was little time for comprehensive primary health care. Consequently, Dixon, Kelly and Kirke recommended that Northern Territory health-workers focus solely on clinical care, and that an Indigenous worker be employed specifically to address broader primary health care issues.

Paradoxically, a report from Western Australia at about the same time[36] advocated a broad approach. It cited more optimistic sources, such as Soong's definition of the healthworker role,[37] doctors' accounts from the Northern Territory programme and supportive international accounts.

The broad conception of healthworker practice was further endorsed by two key publications at the end of the 1980s: *Koorie Health in Koorie Hands*, written by an Aboriginal doctor, and the official *National Aboriginal Health Strategy*.[38] Both promoted Aboriginal control of health service delivery and a broad 'Aboriginal' approach. They emphasised the social, emotional and cultural wellbeing of the whole community—a 'whole of life' view.[39]

The term 'Aboriginal' increasingly signified the service provider as well as the recipient of health services. According to Rose Ellis, then editor of the *Aboriginal and Islander Health Worker Journal*, the broad practice of healthworkers was 'very special':

> Aboriginal and Islander healthworkers hold a *very special* position within their communities which is not to be found in any other area of community health. They are the information brokers, the advisers, the fixers, the health educators, the mental health work-ers, the domestic violence and drug and alcohol counsellors, the housing officers, the police liaison, the translators, the representa-tives and most often the voice of the people they serve.[40]

While the National Aboriginal Health Strategy report endorsed healthworkers undertaking individual and community-focused curative, preventive and promotional practices, it did not specifically conceptu-alise or promote a 'holistic' practice. Following its release, however, both training providers and federal and state governments undertook projects to identify core healthworker competencies in order to develop accredited training courses.[41] These projects led to even broader constructions of healthworker practice, as various health professionals lobbied for the inclusion of their particular specialisation.

Echoing Skeet's observation of Primary Health Workers in the international context,[42] Franks and Curr criticised the unrealistic expectations of Aboriginal healthworkers,

> Treatment of common sicknesses; implementation of preventative programmes; implementation of community education programmes; promotion of environmental sanitation measures; and the management of the Health Centre … At a minimum, these duties represent five positions in a non-Aboriginal organisation.[43]

These authors and others reported that in the context of high clinical morbidity within remote communities in Western Australia and the Northern Territory, most healthworkers worked alongside nurses as their assistants.[44]

Nevertheless, a comprehensive primary health care approach continued to be advocated at higher policy levels, especially within the federal health bureaucracy.[45] Likewise, the Health Department of Western Australia developed a career structure for healthworkers based on a generalist role, and complementary training was formalised.[46]

Paradoxically, the Health Department of Western Australia was at the same time shifting to a funder/purchaser/provider model of health service. Health service providers (for example, an Aboriginal Health Service) now contracted with the purchaser (for example, the Health Department) to deliver particular health services for specific populations.[47] This resulted in the purchasing of 'vertical' programmes focused narrowly on specific interventions and requiring specialist healthworkers—compared with broader primary health care approaches. As one healthworker observed, while many healthworkers were trained and employed as broad generalists, employers often placed them in a specialised area of which they had only superficial knowledge.[48]

Applied research from the Northern Territory indicated that

healthworkers were frustrated and confused, and that the many positive images created by public rhetoric and theory did not translate into practice,[49] as the level of clinical morbidity and the dependence on nurses meant that most healthworkers still worked as clinical assistants. The healthworkers themselves advocated the need for 'holistic' practice.

Healthworkers have always faced divergent conceptions of their practice and of its place in the struggle to improve the health of Aboriginal people. Evidence suggests that several serious problems beset the role of Aboriginal healthworkers.[50] Aboriginal healthworkers predominantly deliver clinical care; health service managers and other health professionals frequently hold disparate views about their role and have little understanding of their training and/or how to work with them; supervision is often ad hoc; many healthworkers work as subordinates; and uncertainty arises among healthworkers when guidelines governing other health professionals circumscribe the scope of their practice. In such circumstances, it is not surprising that resignation rates of healthworkers are high.[51]

The role of the healthworker has evolved in the context of diverse international precedents, contentious professional politics, disparate client needs in both rural and urban settings, and a need for skilful practice both within the clinic and in clients' homes and community settings. Consequently, healthworkers undertake a vast range of tasks and their practice, within efforts to co-ordinate registration and training nationally and to professionalise the role, remains contested.

But how do healthworkers themselves describe and understand their professional practice? This book, located within the Family Care section of an Aboriginal community-controlled health service, is the first detailed ethnographic study of healthworker practice.

THE ABORIGINAL HEALTH SERVICE

The Aboriginal healthworkers at the heart of this book operated from the Family Care section and related domains of an urban Aboriginal Health Service. Aboriginal Health Services are non-government, Aboriginal-controlled organisations that provide health services primarily for Indigenous people. Established nearby in 1973, this AHS operated from a converted 1960s warehouse on a street corner in a mixed commercial and professional part of the city. The Family Care section was on an adjacent corner in a converted 1900s house behind a fast-food outlet. Most of the Aboriginal population in the city once lived in the immediate neighbourhood. However, the renovation of houses for professional and commercial use during the past fifteen years had dispersed most of the Aboriginal tenants, and the city's Aboriginal population of 10,000–12,000 was now scattered throughout the suburbs, within an arc extending 25–30 kilometres from the old neighbourhood.

The AHS is legally incorporated and answerable to an elected Aboriginal council. The executive director, who is a member of the council, is responsible for day-to-day management. At the time of this study in the late 1990s, there were almost 60 staff, over 2000 clients and an operating budget of approximately 1.5 million dollars derived from federal and state government grants, contracts and Medicare payments. Staff worked in sectional teams, which included the Family Care team, Medical Clinic team, Welfare team, Health Promotion team and Administration team (including the Transport section). A team leader managed each section, and the team leaders together constituted a management team, led by the executive director.

The Family Care section was set up in 1988 and is described like this in the corporate plan:

> The Family Care programme provides practical assistance, clinical care and support for Aboriginal people with terminal illnesses or permanent functional disability and their carers. The main aim of the programme is to enable individuals to live in their own home environment with independence, security and dignity for as long as practicable.

The Family Care team leader was the manager of two separate government-funded programmes, Home and Community Care and Chronic Care. Home and Community Care provided weekly home services to 88 frail-aged and disabled clients. Chronic Care provided daily home care to 15 clients. Family Care employed six permanent healthworkers, including a team leader and two relief healthworkers.

They worked alongside a field nurse, a community development officer, a care-aide and a cleaner.

The activities of healthworkers within Family Care included welfare services, clinical monitoring, making appointments, recording client statistics, counselling, organising social visits, personal care assistance, transport, advocacy, referral, rehabilitation support, paramedical assistance, hospital visits, home visits, palliative care, shopping, and liaison with other sections of the AHS and other service providers. Many of their clients had lived in rural areas for the first thirty years of their lives. Most now lived within a 25–30 kilometre radius of the AHS, with clusters in particular areas—and very few drove cars. The primary source of income for most clients was the aged or disability support pension. Most came to Family Care through referrals from other AHS workers.

Table 1 provides a generalised profile of the illnesses and conditions suffered by Family Care clients. Blindness, deafness, gastric ulcers, psychological disabilities and other illnesses associated with ageing were common. In brief, the Family Care healthworkers worked with a group of clients who suffered with many of the clinical as well as social health problems endemic to the Aboriginal community.

The Family Care healthworkers

This book is about the work of ten healthworkers employed in six permanent Family Care positions and four employed in other sections of the AHS. Healthworkers are defined in this study as graduates from a healthworker training course. All participants had undertaken generalist training, full-time for at least one year, with a specialised Aboriginal healthworker training college. One year of training (approximately 40 weeks) covered Aboriginal Studies (history and culture), Epidemiology (determining priorities and prevention strategies), Environmental Health (water supply, housing and sanitation), Health Promotion (design, implementation and evaluation), Human Biology (bodily systems), Applied Health Management (assessment, basic treatments, referral and programme management), Alcohol and Drug Issues (assessment and counselling), Mental Health (assessment, advocacy and medications),

TABLE 1: Health Conditions Affecting Family Care Clients (n = 103)

Condition	Percentage affected
Diabetes (types 1 and 2)	53
Hypertension	49
Heart disease	38
Arthritis	31
Asthma	27
Obesity	24
Renal disease	18

Sexuality and Health (screening, STD tracing and control), Medications (protocols, effects, administration and precautions), Maternal and Child Health (antenatal care, child development and childhood illnesses) and a placement for six weeks in a clinical setting.[52] In its early days the college was a part of the AHS and some on-the-job training was available. The training also included field visits and placements of up to one week with other agencies. Some healthworkers had further qualifications: three had a university degree in Indigenous Community Health and four had previously worked in hospitals as enrolled nurses or as nursing assistants.

The following chapters provide insight into the everyday world of Aboriginal healthworkers. In the marginalised context of their day-to-day delivery of services to clients and their work alongside other health professionals, many of the assumptions, principles and ideals underpinning Indigenous healthworker practice are brought into question. By highlighting that experience and knowledge, and by bringing the voices of Aboriginal healthworkers to the foreground, my intent is to show how disruptions to their practice occur and to compare those findings with the existing literature about healthworker practice.

Grassroots Healthworker Practice

Myriad demands and pressures mark the day-to-day practice of the Family Care Aboriginal healthworkers. They arise from the social exclusion and poverty experienced by many Aboriginal people and, in particular, from ongoing crises within contemporary Aboriginal families.

Potentially, healthworkers can provide their clients with access to health care services, housing support, transport, financial assistance and advocacy. As a result, clients place wide-ranging demands upon them. Likewise, claims on healthworkers emerge from other health professionals, who seek to engage them as assistants. History also plays a role in the delivery of prescribed medical care within the Aboriginal community. The everyday currency of stories of historical neglect and abuse passed down within the community is yet another challenge to health care provision. The following stories present the realities of grassroots healthworker practice. A frank account emerges of these healthworkers, both as Aboriginal people and as health professionals.

In the first part of this chapter, Rita describes the broad parameters of healthworker practice and its associated pressures. Next, Rose, the team leader of Family Care, highlights the complexities of practice beset by circumstances of exclusion and poverty. Finally, June identifies the critical concerns confronting healthworkers engaged with Aboriginal families today.

DIVERSE DEMANDS, MULTIPLE DILEMMAS

'A Jack of all trades'

Rita finds that client activities often conflict with the plans of health-workers. In her experience, client priorities that relate to immediate social needs distract attention from clinical monitoring and other preventive practices. Rita knows that client need, met without careful thought, can foster dependency, and she is also aware of the vulnerability of healthworkers to co-option by other professionals. Her perception is that the combination of these factors results in healthworkers being over-stretched.

In her mid-thirties, Rita grew up with her family in a rural town. She completed Year Eleven at school, and in her early twenties completed healthworker training. Having finished the course, the only job she could get in the health arena was as a speech therapist's assistant at the district hospital. She later moved to the city and worked in a variety of administrative positions before joining Family Care.

Rita voices her concerns in a discussion among healthworkers about home visits. She had spent all that day in court, waiting to give evidence for a client facing eviction from her home. She expresses not only her frustration at 'wasting' another day in court, but also her feelings of guilt towards other clients who, in her absence, missed out on a home visit. In her disquiet, she uses the forum to challenge various facets of healthworker practice:

> I reckon we create dependency ... I'm not a lawyer, and I've been spending all week at court. I'm not a lawyer, I'm a healthworker— and I feel like everything that I've learnt, like all the paramedical stuff, that's not important! It's all the social stuff—I feel like the social takes over, more than the paramedical or anything to do with medical ... Like I can see the point of someone going with them [to court]—it's just that it seems it is always the healthworker, and it should be the family, or even Welfare's job ... Health-workers—see this is what I mean—it's like the Jack of all trades ... when you are doing all these other things ... there's not enough of you.

Rita's outburst reveals crucial elements of her experience as a healthworker. Within the philosophy of holistic service provision, she feels besieged and pulled in competing directions by the multiple demands of her frail-aged and disabled clients. Rita believes that a healthworker should provide predominantly clinical or 'paramedical' services. Instead, she finds herself burdened with myriad social welfare services. Rita fears that healthworkers foster dependency by servicing clients' broad social needs. Not only does she feel over-stretched by these needs, but her work is subject to directives from health professionals and managers outside the Family Care section where she works.

'The social takes over the paramedical'

Despite Rita's emphasis on clinical duties, she is well aware of the widespread social needs in her community and believes she must address the legacies of enforced family separation, social exclusion, cultural oppression and racism suffered by many of her frail-aged clients. Many have a history of mistreatment, hardship and family separations. Most grew up and lived through the oppression of the Aborigines Act 1905 from the 1940s to the 1960s,[1] and the subsequent paternalistic assimilation era.

Rita knows that establishing new relationships and placing trust in strangers is perceived by clients as threatening and unsafe. Along with this mistrust goes an unwillingness among the elderly clients to seek care, and a view of service providers as threatening. She considers that a major part of her work stems from their lack of confidence in dealing with non-Aboriginal health professionals:

> A healthworker is a person who has medical skills and is a link between the professional people like doctors and nurses, and all those sorts of professional people, to the Aboriginal community. Like, if we're talking about Aboriginal healthworkers, I think we're sort of like the middleman—'cause I mean, they're our people. We know how to deal with our own people. It's easier for our clients to talk to us rather than professionals like doctors and nurses and all that sort of stuff, and we have a lot of medical sort of background—and not only medical but there's a lot of welfare stuff.

Like, most of our clients are elderly and I think, because in their young life they were involved with assimilation and getting taken away from their parents and taken into mission-type places, they got a lot of self-esteem taken off them. Their language—they weren't allowed to speak their language, it was *shame** to talk the language and that sort of stuff, and I think that has filtered through today. So they're not very confident, our elderly people, because— I'm not saying all, but most of the oldies that I've met—they *shame*. 'Cause they've gone through all that, and they find that non-Aboriginal people are threatening and they can't really talk to them.

We are Aboriginal—and I find it, and they find it, much easier to talk to us if they've got a problem, because they probably know that we've been through something like that, that they went through—like racism and that sort of stuff … Them old fellas, they like to get on and not worry about it, and cause a problem because they think they're gonna be a pain in the butt or something … Maybe because of that history they're not very confident with saying, 'I've got something wrong, I feel dizzy'. The whole problem could be diabetes, but they just fob it off because, 'Oh well, no one wants to know, and I don't want to be a pain', and that sort of attitude. So I think it's good that we have a link—we're the middleman, that sort of thing.

The healthworkers provide a necessary and comprehensive link between their marginalised clients and a broad array of health services, both those they provide themselves and more complex services from other professionals and agencies. Rita links her clients to these services by providing transport and advocacy—for example, by taking a client to court and giving evidence to prevent her eviction.

---

*An Aboriginal-English expression used here to mean, in broad terms, unacceptable or shameful.

Although Rita feels both upset and guilty about her court advocacy duties compromising her services to other clients, her healthworker colleagues endorse her court attendance, particularly the advocacy and the emotional support:

> **Ruby**: If you're going to be holistic then ... you have to address the client's priorities. I mean, I hate sitting in court, I think it's a big waste of time and I hate doing it after a while, but you just have to do it.
>
> **Rita**: Well, when you're neglecting [the other clients] and they ring up and say, 'Where you been?', y'know, you feel terrible.
>
> **Merle**: We spent the whole afternoon [in court]—the whole day really.
>
> **Patty**: And then they had a closed court.
>
> **Ruby**: For a client it's a great support because they feel comfortable with you.
>
> **Merle**: That's right.
>
> **Rita**: I know for Tootsie, she felt comfortable when I was with her—just having another Aboriginal person around.
>
> **June**: Yeah.

While Rita acknowledges the value of her advocacy, and in particular its emotional support component, she is perturbed that the social dimension of client need takes precedence over paramedical need. Her training emphasised a more clinical definition of the healthworker role:

> I don't expect it to be all paramedical, but that would be more a priority for a healthworker ... I just feel that we do a lot of, a lot of social stuff ... I just think—what I'm getting at is the whole training you get as a healthworker has got [nothing] to do with the hands-on job ... I was trained in the early stages of the whole healthworker programme, and a lot of it was clinical—there was a bit of social, but most of it was clinical—and that's how I've always thought as a healthworker.

In practice, clients without food, clothing and shelter confront Rita:

> There's a lot of welfare stuff, and I reckon we deal more with the social welfare stuff than actually going out doing blood pressures and sugar levels and medications and that sort of thing. In my experience, I think we do a lot of welfare stuff—things like getting housing, getting food for the families.

The healthworkers report that when approaching a client's front door, they must be prepared to expect anything:

> **June**: The first thing you think about as you pull up in the drive is, 'What am I gonna get today?'
>
> **Ruby**: That's the trouble with home visits—you can't plan the home visit 'cause you don't know what's going to happen until you get to that house.
>
> **Rita**: Yep.
>
> **Ruby**: So you can't have a standard or you can't plan the home visits. When you walk in that door, anything could happen … you just never know. Some days I pray that no one's home.

Home visits are unpredictable, and healthworkers confront varying and indeterminate needs. This is partly because many frail-aged clients are twenty years younger than their non-Aboriginal counterparts. They hold a range of family responsibilities and are often still socially active.

Josie, a fellow healthworker, illustrates the complexity produced by the fusion of social and clinical need:

> This lady is constantly in need. She's got high blood pressure, she can't handle her money. I've been taking her to welfare place, getting food hampers, clothes. I've even been with her shopping to see how she spends her money to try and help her. She smokes a lot. We need someone to work out a budget with her, we've tried it ourselves. We need a full-on thing with her—she doesn't have enough money for medication. I've been ringing around for her

bills, trying to get extensions. Her son's in prison—we take her there, but now he's been transferred to [a rural prison] and she wants us to take her there. There's lots of family problems—her de facto is a drunk and is always abusing her, there's people coming over and drinking, she's got no way of getting round. We've tried to get her involved in some day outings, but she's not really interested.

While Josie desperately juggles her client's multiple social and clinical needs, Joan, a Family Care care-aide, services a client whose 'social' problems appear more psychosocial:

The other lady I see is very demanding. She's very subtle about it … I feel, I just feel exhausted—I do. She's just measly. I feel, wow, I've never met anyone like her. She can mentally just wear you down—incredible. She is so gentle—honestly, it's just incredible, and yet she will get away with it all the time … almost like an addiction. I find with her, she's got to have something free given to her all the time. She's got to go back with something that's given to her. (giggles) It's true—whether it be money, or even if she goes to a second-hand shop and gets something, or if she can book up something, she's got to come back with something … Her cupboard's stocked up with food and everything, yet she's still able to go up to the relief-for-food place, and she still comes home with something … I feel very wrong about it actually, I really do. I think it's not right because it feels like—she is just getting, like it's a greed.

This client's psychosocial problems and Joan's involvement in their resolution causes her to question her own ethics and values.

The confluence of clinical and social need means that apparently simple tasks become complicated and time consuming. Sometimes the transportation of a client becomes messy, as Merle illustrates:

With Mimi—like, last Thursday she had to come in to see Glenda [the Welfare section social worker]. I'd rung her and said, 'I will be there by eight-thirty and I'll bring you in with me when I come to work'. Well I had to wait—actually I got there at eight o'clock—they weren't ready till nine … I [also] had to pick someone else up and bring her in to the dentist. So all these kids wanted to come too, in the car—Mimi's grandkids, two of them, and Fred, and her—so there's five in the car … So I had to come [to the AHS] and drop them off and then go to Newtown and pick [the other client] up.

Merle feels an obligation to consider not only transport for Mimi but also child-care for her grandchildren. However, this interferes with her initial plans.

When taking a holistic approach to service provision, healthworkers can face complex cases where clinical, social and psychosocial factors intersect. These cases require high levels of interpretation and judgement and constitute a major demand on their time and skills.

However, interventions can be more straightforward. A paramedical approach confines the task to a narrow, clinical set of duties, which includes assessing a client's physical wellbeing, monitoring blood pressures and blood sugar levels, ensuring medication supplies and dressing wounds. Rita reports that a narrow, clinical approach is often all a client wants. 'See, if the family's there, like all the family, most people want you to do what you have to do—and get out!' A narrow clinical approach is also an option or even a 'way out' when healthworkers feel pressured in their work.

While Rita is distressed about the primacy of social issues over paramedical issues, she finds that when her practice does focus consistently on the paramedical, this paradoxically creates a tension. She reports that a constant narrow clinical focus creates unsatisfying, boring work:

I think that it's a monotonous job. Everyday it's the same clients, the same job, the same routine. Some of the girls have been there for five years or more and I just can't understand how—that's me personally, I would just become brain-dead because of the repetitiveness of the job … I was employed as a relief, and, like, I've been here nearly five months straight and it gets really boring. Like the job—y'know what I mean—it's a job that you do every day, the same thing, and I think—that's what it is for me anyway.

In response, Rose outlines her expectations of healthworker practice:

> You're supposed to work with your client, and work out programmes with your client. Now if it is boring for you it's because … you're not actually doing what you're supposed to be doing, which is talking to your client, working out with your client what you could be doing for them … Like a diabetic—get involved with them, work on a programme, and saying:
>
>> Look, I'm coming to visit you every Wednesday. On this Wednesday I'll have two maybe three hours with you. I can allow that much time with you. We can either go to the diabetic clinic and buy you all the stuff that you need (if they need syringes or if they need blood sticks) or we can go for a walk in the park. We can go and have a cup of tea.
>
> That time is allowed for that client. At the moment the healthworkers are just going out, seeing the client, doing their blood sugar, blood pressure and walking out the door. Now if you do that every day, I'd be bored to tears too.

The response to Rose from some healthworkers indicates that such efforts are often fruitless:

> **Merle**: A lot of the clients don't want to do that.
> **June**: A lot of them don't like leaving their place.
> **Rita**: They've got no self-determination themselves … I think a lot of clients are just happy with what we are giving them, as long as they're getting their sugar done, and their blood pressure and their medications. 'Cause, y'know, sometimes I've offered some of our oldies, when it's hot, 'Do you want to go down to the beach, or go for a drive along the coast?' 'Oh no, no!' You're right—y'know a lot of them just don't have the energy … when

they're sick and old and that, they just want to sit home, y'know what I mean, and that's where they're comfortable.

Merle (laughing): None of my clients want to go anywhere except Mavis … and they won't walk, Rose, they won't walk anywhere. *Who wants to go for a walk?* … Like Phyllis, I went there one day and she wanted to go to the park. I said, 'Well we'll all go to the park—I'll take you and the kids'. And then she said, 'Well we better not, because [the parents] might come back looking for the kids'.

The healthworkers find that preventive activities are difficult to arrange when clients do not have a telephone, lack sufficient energy or interest, have responsibilities for grandchildren or are simply more comfortable staying at home. Moreover, they report that clients do not see such activities as part of the healthworker role.

However, Rose responds that clients need to be educated about the realities of health prevention practices:

Rose: We need to get through to the clients that taking a blood pressure is not really improving their health. They need to be looking at all these other factors—to include their health in their lifestyle. I mean, we can go out and take their blood pressure ten times a day—their health's not going to improve. You can go out there and instead of walking in, doing their blood pressure, blood sugar level, maybe checking their tablets, then walking out the door, you need to sit there and check them—say, 'Look, we need to talk about your problems, these are the things we need to be looking at'.

Ruby: Well, maybe if their sugar is high, say to them, 'Next Tuesday, I'll pick you up and we'll go shopping together. Let's shop properly. I'll explain which [foods] are good, and which are not good', y'know—or do it over a couple of weeks.

Despite feedback from their colleagues, Ruby and Rose each maintain a vision of an ideal intervention linked to a holistic philosophy of service provision. They envisage that during home visits, healthworkers will establish and maintain a dialogue with the client about healthy behaviours and, ideally, actively engage the client in walking or shopping for healthy foods. Within this holistic mode, tension exists not only between social and paramedical needs, but also between healthworker and client priorities. Clients often resist engagement in preventive health practices.

A common experience is that the immediate context determines what takes place on a home visit. A narrow clinical approach may be taken when the healthworker is busy, the client is indifferent to her presence or the family is at home. A more holistic approach is possible if the healthworker has the time and the client is responsive. However, healthworkers often find themselves acting as middleman—addressing immediate social needs such as food shortages, financial shortfalls and housing issues.

'Colleagues don't see our case load as important'

Healthworkers find that their role as a middleman attracts the interest of other health professionals within the health service. Rita recognises the necessity of being a middleman, and her clients' need for both advocacy and emotional support. However, she questions why it is 'always provided by the healthworker'. Reflecting on her attendance at court, she proposes that such work is the duty of a welfare worker:

> I don't know why the Welfare section weren't there. I asked the welfare assistant. He would do it, but those other people in Welfare, they get him to do other things that are more important to them—they don't think a healthworker's caseload is important.

Rita suggests that some senior workers in the AHS Welfare section fail to recognise the work commitments of the Family Care healthworkers. In her view, they attempt to co-opt healthworkers to service welfare needs, and this explains her attendance at court. However, Ruby informs Rita that a healthworker is necessary in the court due to legal and bureaucratic requirements: 'They need the service provider there so you can say what service you provide, what services they need—only the person providing the service can do that'.

It is true that in eviction cases, like this one, only evidence from a person directly providing services to the client in the home is admissible to the court.

Nonetheless, given the demands of Family Care duties, Rita remains disconcerted by the expectation that healthworkers will comply with requests of other AHS health professionals. She reports that the request for her to attend court originated from a social worker in the Welfare section:

> Glenda [the social worker] rang me and said, 'Would you be able to come with Tootsie [to the court]? Can you pick her up?' So I said, 'Yeah, no worries', and I picked her up. And that was it—I was involved.

Rita perceives herself as a Jack of all trades who provides holistic services not only to clients of Family Care, but also to other health professionals in the AHS.

Her colleagues have similar concerns. They query the right of a social worker in the Welfare section to request Rita to undertake court work. They detect that within the AHS a perception exists that healthworkers are available as junior assistants. For instance, June reports that a Welfare social worker suggested she assist a Welfare client to move house. June's indignation emerges in her response:

> **June**: She's wanting me to go out, clean, wash, scrub and all.
> **Merle**: I wouldn't do that.
> **June**: And whatever—pack, transport her and all her belongings and her husband, a strong healthy man who can't do a thing at home … She wants me to go out. Welfare just rang me up to see if I can transport them or whatever. I'll tell you for a fact, when I worked in Welfare for seven years I done that myself there in that position, and I don't think a healthworker should lower their grade to go down to do it.

June is unwilling to undertake the work duties of a welfare worker. She perceives such work as beneath a healthworker. Her response suggests that she attaches considerable status to her healthworker role.

According to Ruby, AHS welfare workers and doctors often, without prior consultation, make client appointments that implicate healthworkers:

> The trouble comes when the appointments are made out of your hands—like when [the social worker] makes the appointment, the doctors make the appointment. 'Cause they make the appointment regardless of what your time [schedule] is … Or they'll give the appointment card to the client thinking that the client's going to tell their healthworker—and then that client will see you next visit and will say, 'I'm supposed to be here today. Can you take me?'

Healthworkers also have transport obligations. Because they use an AHS vehicle, AHS procedures oblige them to undertake transport duties at the direction of the transport manager:

> **Merle**: If [the Transport section] want us—y'know.
> **Joan**: And we're not busy … if we are finished our day's work.
> **Ruby**: They can even ring us in the field and say, 'Such and such needs to be picked up—where are you?' … Now if you're in that area, you gotta leave your client and do the transport.
> **Joan**: If it's convenient.

In balancing the competing demands of clients, doctors, social workers and the transport manager, Rita finds that her capacity as a healthworker is stretched to the point where there is 'not enough of you'.

'She wants my life'

Rita perceives that when healthworkers cater to broad social welfare needs, clients become dependent and less reliant on utilising their own resources. In this respect, transport is central. Clients perceive Rita as a potential taxi-driver. She receives requests for an array of transport services, such as conveying client washing to another relative's house, undertaking shopping expeditions and transporting grandchildren. By acquiescing to such requests, Rita believes that healthworkers foster dependency.

Negotiating client requests is difficult for Rita. She recounts that since accompanying Tootsie to court, which in itself compromised other client services, Tootsie has made even greater claims:

> I went to pick her up this morning and she was still in the shower, and she told me to go on … Ever since the court, being involved with the court and that … she's dependent … I don't mind pickin' up Tootsie, she's just round the corner, but she's really depending on me a lot now, since the court case and that. She's too much … she wants everything—medication, my life, courier, pick up things … Not only that—because she is linked with my family, y'know, she thinks, 'Oh y'know, you're our family'. You're obligated in that way … That's why I do think we create a lot of dependency here … She uses me, too … so she's become a bit of a problem for me.

In short, Rita perceives that Tootsie is a problem because she has become dependent. Her family tie to Tootsie further complicates matters. Rita feels compelled to assist because of family obligations, especially since Tootsie is older. (In similar instances within Family Care, the team leader has re-assigned the caseload to another healthworker.)

Rita cites another example of dependency: when clients telephone her at the AHS and ask her to make appointments:

> There's a lot of dependency … To try and get people out of that is really hard—I mean, you've got clients ringing up here saying, 'Oh can you ring up and make an appointment for me for rah rah rah?' Now they just used thirty cents to ring you to make the appointment when they could just ring straight through. They know you're there to do it, y'know what I mean, and you think, 'Why didn't you just ring straight through to AHS and make the appointment yourself?'

Dependency is also a problem in relation to the supply of medications by the AHS. Following medical consultations, doctors give clients an initial prescription free of charge and a swatch of repeat prescriptions that they must pay a pharmacist to supply. Nevertheless, instead of filling a repeat script, clients often ring the AHS and request a new prescription, knowing they will incur no charge. In a Family Care meeting, Rita and Josie recognise the need to carefully discriminate between such requests:

> **Josie**: You shouldn't have clients where they get it [free] anyway—
> every time they need medication. They become dependent on
> it. 'Oh yeah, pick us up something from the chemist', it
> becomes a regular thing—only when they need it.
> **Rita**: Yeah, I watch mine.
> **Josie**: It's becoming a regular thing … only when they need it.
> **Rita**: Only when they're really desperate and they've got no money.
> **Josie**: Say in an off-pension week when they've got no money.
> **Rita**: That's right.

Quoting an instance when a doctor accompanied her on a home visit, Josie indicates that some doctors encourage such dependency:

> Because I notice with the doctors, they encourage us to bring the
> scripts back to the AHS pharmacist. Like with the doctor today,
> she went out to a client and she said, 'Do you want Josie to take
> the script back and get it filled for you?' And I was like, I'm trying
> to tell her, 'No, I'm sorry'—because I think the client should fill
> the script herself.

Healthworkers face a bewildering challenge—to discourage dependency while working within a holistic practice framework. A holistic practice within a context of constant need leaves them vulnerable to wide-ranging demands which, from their viewpoint, will foster dependency if met. This situation challenges their ability both to discriminate and to negotiate 'legitimate' needs. While Rita clearly recognises the special needs of her clients, she feels vulnerable to acquiescing to unreasonable demands, particularly in the absence of formal guidelines governing a holistic approach.

'Not enough of you'

Family Care healthworkers service frail-aged and elderly clients who share a history of family separation, social exclusion, cultural oppression and racism. Consequently, many have little self-esteem, perceive non-Aboriginal health and welfare professionals as threatening, and lack the self-confidence to engage them. Healthworkers perceive that they play an important role both as a non-threatening provider of health care and as an agent for their clients' dealings with non-Aboriginal health professionals. They perceive the clients as 'our people' and empathise deeply with their concerns. However, in such a demanding context, this sentiment occasions situations where they can become overwhelmed—for instance, by attending to one client's needs to the detriment of another.

The team leader encourages healthworkers to engage in preventive programmes, such as exercising with clients or demonstrating healthy shopping practices. However, clients resist such attempts. Only occasionally do they wish to go out, because they are responsible for looking after grandchildren or do not see the provision of excursions as a healthworker's task. If clients have family present or particular personal priorities, they are unwilling to engage in extended consultations during home visits. While ready to seek a healthworker's assistance to meet their own definition of need, they are frequently less accommodating of the healthworkers' preventive health priorities.

Healthworkers encounter numerous demands to advocate on their clients' behalf in relation to social problems—housing, income support, inadequate food supplies and a lack of transport. As the immediate short-term agendas of the client frequently take precedence, the social is often a larger component of the work than the paramedical. The social also encompasses the psychosocial. Due to the emphasis on clinical aspects of health during training, and her designation as a *health* worker, Rita questions whether it should always be the healthworker attending to these taxing social concerns.

Additional obligations increase the burden. Despite having a caseload of clients whose needs are exacting, professionals from other sections of the AHS often co-opt healthworkers. Pulled in multiple directions, a healthworker can feel like a Jack of all trades.

Healthworkers find the holistic approach encourages ambit claims upon their services by other staff and by clients. The philosophy within Family Care is to encourage clients to 'take control' of their lives. While most healthworkers can discern legitimate needs within ambit claims, they often lack the requisite skills to negotiate with clients and, by acquiescing to inessential demands, they feel they encourage dependent behaviours. Policies such as the provision of free medications also undermine attempts to challenge dependency. Subject to the broad demands from both clients and other staff, Rita feels there is simply 'not enough of you'. Dependency of clients is a major concern for all the healthworkers within Family Care.

A DISPIRITED RESPONSE

'You feel, what's the point'

Although she herself is Aboriginal, Rose experiences difficulty engaging the trust of clients. She perceives that they transfer their mistrust and fear of non-Aboriginal health professionals onto Aboriginal healthworkers. She and her colleagues direct considerable effort towards winning client trust but, nonetheless, many fail to maintain medication schedules or respond to health education. Unsurprisingly, many healthworkers experience deep frustration in the face of such unrewarding responses. Rose perceives that in addition to fear and mistrust, social factors such as poverty, inadequate housing and a lack of education are major determinants of client ill health. She recognises that most of these factors are beyond healthworker control.

Within Family Care, Rose supervises nine staff and manages both the Home and Community Care programme and the Chronic Care programme. The capacity to take responsibility came early in Rose's life. She grew up in a small country town, 150 kilometres north of the city. When she was a ten-year-old schoolgirl, her mother died. As the eldest daughter of a large family, Rose left school to care for her siblings.

After working as a nursing assistant in country hospitals, Rose moved to the city and worked first in a large geriatric hospital and later in a children's hospital, where she completed eighteen months of hospital-based nursing training. After securing work at the AHS, Rose completed an Advanced Certificate in Aboriginal Health from the Aboriginal Health-worker Training College, followed by a university degree in Indigenous Community Health. She has been an AHS healthworker for nine years.

Rose narrates her healthworker experiences while sitting in her office, which overlooks the street opposite the entrance of the main AHS building. Above the entrance, a heavy metal roller-door hangs like a steel curtain. Through the window, the painted brick of the double-storey, flat-roofed converted warehouse appears dulled by the atmos-phere of the inner city. Outside, people sit in parked cars or bend over car windows. Family members stand in small groups or squat on the pavement, some yarning, some smoking and watching the street. The fast-food outlet on the corner receives a constant trickle of clients. Children boisterously taunt and shriek, and an elderly client shuffles across the street. We hear the client complaining at the front desk, her voice competing with the constant demand of the telephone.

Rose faces a continuing and difficult dilemma: how to manage a programme that, in her view, is unable to consistently achieve healthy outcomes for the clients. In a candid and defining moment, she expresses her despair at the seeming pointlessness of healthworker inter-ventions in the face of massive social problems:

> When I was going out in the field I found it really difficult to start with. It was just sort of getting to know the people and getting their trust. You sort of feel like you are just doing a sort of bandaid treatment out there. You're just going out there and doing the same things day in and day out with no improvement—nothing is happening … You're going out there telling everyone to take their medication, it's going to get better, if you do this it's going to get better—but it doesn't seem to get better … Sometimes you feel, what's the point—there doesn't seem to be any point in it … Why am I doing it? The main hassle is the fact that it is the same problems—they don't go away.

Rose's candour reveals a set of core practice issues: 1) problems gaining the trust of clients; 2) difficulties convincing clients to engage with medication schedules and health-enhancing behaviours; 3) constant encounters with endemic social problems which engulf clients and dwarf healthworker efforts; and 4) a constant wrestle with an underlying feeling of despair at the apparent lack of client progress.

'It's difficult getting their trust'

Rose echoes Rita's perception of a reluctance among clients to seek care, which Rita attributes to the mistreatment and hardship suffered by that generation. In Rose's experience many clients fear and mistrust strangers. 'I found it really difficult to start with—it was just sort of getting to know the people and getting their trust', she said.

Other healthworkers agree. According to Margie, 'You have to earn a patient's trust—if they don't trust you they won't let you in the front door. As you build the trust they feel more confident with you.' Christine describes the beginning of a relationship with one of her clients:

> His name was Dodger … With Aboriginal people, it takes them a while to build up their trust in you—once they build up their trust in you, you're right … The first day he wouldn't say much to me, and I'd say, 'C'mon Dodger—I'm like you, I'm Aboriginal', and then he'd say, 'Oh yeah, I'll teach you some language', and he started teaching me bird names.

Over time, healthworkers generally gain some level of trust with clients, but clients often remain mistrustful of doctors and hospitals:

> They hate hospitals…you wouldn't get many of them to a doctor. As I said, it takes a while to build up a relationship when they first see you. A lot of people, when they're sick they won't tell you. A lot of the real old ones, they'd just rather lay down and die—it's sad … I don't think they like hospitals—they hate hospitals … You wouldn't get many of them to a doctor—they have to be dragged there.

A home visit to Christine's client Reggie highlights this reluctance. He lives in a Government Housing Commission unit adjacent to the freeway. During the visit, Reggie sits at the table in the living room while his daughter cooks in the kitchen. A baby is asleep on the sofa. Six other grandchildren between the ages of two and seven watch television, wrestle, come and go from the kitchen and gather around Christine. As Christine informs Reggie of his doctor's appointment, his daughter overhears the conversation:

> **Christine**: Your [doctor's] appointment is in the book for the Transport [the AHS driver] to come and get you.
> **Daughter**: *Now, you've got no excuse!*

The daughter's comment suggests that Reggie is prone to use any available excuse to avoid seeing the doctor.

As suggested by Rita, healthworkers attempt to overcome client mistrust of other health professionals by providing emotional support and by advocating for clients at their appointments. In a discussion concerning the treatment of clients in hospitals, Ruby outlines how a healthworker can help overcoming misunderstandings:

> See, a lot of family too, they don't feel comfortable in hospitals, and they don't understand what the doctor is saying anyway, a lot of them. So they'd prefer that you went, and you could tell the patient what's going on, and then you can come back to the family and tell them what's happening … Otherwise the family takes them [to hospital], the family doesn't say something—y'know what I mean—'cause they're scared of the hospital themselves. So they go in there, and they see the doctor, and they agree with everything, and then they come home.

'Because I feel good today, I don't need the tablets any more'

Fear and mistrust are major factors not only in relationships between clients and mainstream health professionals, but also in those with

Aboriginal healthworkers. Scepticism is apparent in the half-hearted responses to healthworker attempts to convince clients to adhere to medication schedules.

Building a trusting relationship with clients is difficult enough, according to Rose, but convincing them to adhere to medication schedules and to modify unhealthy behaviours is a formidable task:

> [The clients] think, because they have taken their tablets today and they feel well, that come tomorrow they don't have to take it … They need to take their tablets every day. [They think]— 'because I feel good today, I don't need the tablets any more, so I go off them'—not realising the importance of them.

Likewise, Ruby has trouble convincing her clients to comply with medication regimes,

> Like this client, if she wakes up in the morning, she thinks, 'Oh well, I feel alright, my blood pressure's alright, my sugar level's alright'—then she won't take her tablets … One old lady who has got a urine infection has read somewhere that antibiotics is bad for your body, so she refuses to take them. It's hard for us, 'cause the doctor tells us to make them take their tablets … It doesn't matter how hard we try, if they don't want to take them, they don't want to take them … I persuaded her to take them and she had an adverse reaction—she got cold shivers, really severe aches—so now she is convinced, and now I don't stand a chance of convincing her to take another type … Even some things that aren't related, they'll say, 'Oh that's the tablets'. They've just associated it with the tablets.

Healthworkers observe that many clients mistrust not only health institutions and health professionals, but also their information and remedies, and they place almost as much value on anecdotal evidence as on biomedical knowledge.

The consistent, careful self-management of medications for chronic health conditions is a challenge for many clients. For example, when

Margie asked one client if she had been taking her tablets, the client replied, 'Oh, I'm up and down with them'. When Christine was attending an elderly female client, the son-in-law wandered in from another room. He complained about sore feet, saying they 'really hurt at night'. When questioned whether he self-monitored his blood sugar level, he responded idiosyncratically, 'I don't want to constantly put holes in my fingers'. His mother-in-law then told Christine that his brother had already lost one leg and his mother two legs, from diabetes. Clearly the mother-in-law, who did manage her medication consistently, was becoming an advocate for biomedicine:

> A fella come 'round the other night to visit, who could hardly hold a cup of tea he was shaking so much. I said, 'You should get tablets for that shaking—they've got tablets that can fix that'.

These examples indicate that the notion of tablets as a curative quick-fix is common among clients. However, this notion disrupts secondary prevention treatments that require consistent daily medication. Consequently, healthworkers see little improvement in the wellbeing of such clients, who remain unconvinced about the benefits of maintaining a regimen of prescription drugs and unmoved by health education messages.

'I've talked with her till I'm blue in the face'

During a discussion on delivering health education, the healthworkers report that many clients are unresponsive to their messages. June describes her experiences with Teddy:

> Teddy's into Diet Coke and I'm forever saying, 'You're not supposed to have Diet Coke!' 'But I get high on it—I can get charged up',—I said, you gotta do this and you gotta do that—I was telling him before, but he wouldn't listen. I said, 'Before long, you're going to have a foot, a thumb, a toe or a finger or something cut off', and he wouldn't listen. I went and seen him yesterday [in hospital, after an amputation].

June reports further attempts to educate Teddy, and Merle suggests that smoking could be his problem. When asked how they react to clients who are smokers, the healthworkers respond:

Merle: It's going to kill you Teddy.

June: I usually just say, 'Look, I think you're having one too many. Cut down every day'. The packets they buy are fifty in a packet—the *Holiday* packet.

Josie: They just keep smokin' until there's nothing in it! … We've had times where clients are asking us to take them down the shop to get a packet of smokes! It's like Pauline—she'll say, 'Can you take me down here?' I said, 'Look, I'll take you to the chemist, or whatever else you want to do, but if you just going down there for a packet of smokes, I'm actually encouraging or supporting your habit'. I didn't.

Josie (demonstrating Pauline chain-smoking): Her hand never go down, or have a rest, or anything.

June: And she'll light another one up off that butt!

Josie: Yeah.

Joan: Yeah.

Josie: I've talked with her till I'm blue in the face.

Rita gives another example of what she feels is an unproductive attempt at educating a client:

I've got one client who's heading in for renal failure. She's got a craving for tinned peaches. She's not allowed to have tinned peaches, 'cause it's got so much sugar in it. I said, 'Don't you get the diabetic one?' [She said], '*No way!—Give me the full!*' Y'know, otherwise she don't want it! Y'know, there's little things like that— amazing … [clients] don't even look after themselves. It's really hard to try and get people to get into that way of thinking.

'They never get any better'

While it takes Rose and the other healthworkers a long time to establish trusting relationships with many clients, this alone is not enough. It also takes considerable time and effort to convince clients about appropriate management of their health problems—for instance, to maintain a constant, daily medication regime. Clients who place substantial trust in other sources of information make this even more difficult. They seem to equate medications with cure rather than prevention, and manage their illnesses accordingly. Consequently, healthworkers see little response to their health messages and little improvement in client health:

Josie: [The clients] never get discharged from Family Care—it always continues on and on until either they die or they move, or something like that. It's never because they come good and, y'know, do it on their own and make it and come good, and where we are out doing ourselves out of a job because they're getting better. That's frustrating for me.

Joan: Ongoing.

Josie: Either deaths, or they've moved, or they're on hold, or they've come back and …

Rita: Y'know what—like I think going out and seeing our clients and that, I feel like they never get any better.

June: Yeah.

Merle: Yeah, that's what we're talking about.

Joan: That's what she's saying, there's no progress.

Josie: It's like a never-ending story.

Rita: You don't see someone looking fantastic after, y'know, givin' them the medication, monitoring their blood pressure and …

Josie: That whole idea, y'know, of do ourselves out of a job—and you'd like them just to get above it all.

Rita: It's just like a vicious circle. You're nearly making it, but then something's happened to bring them back, like you said—whether it be death or getting a new house. An endless battle …

Rose's sense of despair about the clients' lack of progress is a common experience for her colleagues. Suggestions that 'they never get any better', 'it's like a never-ending story' or 'an endless battle' indicate that they also share a sense of disillusionment about the work.

'The last thing they think about is their health'

Merle, a recently qualified healthworker with a nursing assistant background, finds the unenthusiastic response of clients deeply frustrating. Her novice status differs from that of her fellow healthworkers, who have all worked for a number of years within either Family Care or other sections of the AHS. In contrast, Merle's previous employment was within mainstream hospitals and nursing homes. Her background is also different: she grew up interstate and has few links to the local Aboriginal community.

In a discussion about the difficulties of safeguarding the health of clients Merle, in a frank and defining moment, shares her deep frustration:

> These people just want to die, they've got a death wish—truly …
> [Phyllis's] legs have swollen up. I don't know how many times I've
> told her to put her feet up when she's sitting down. She drinks at
> home—she reckons she doesn't, but I've noticed her. The last thing
> they think about is their health anyway … Phyllis is always
> worried about her phone, people using her phone! Because if she
> goes off somewhere, she takes the phone with her … [And] there's
> Mickey. He went up bush for a family gathering and what did he
> do? He got drunk, didn't he? I mean, he's on dialysis. So when he
> said that to me, I said, 'Well Mickey, if you get sick, it's your own
> fault' … that's what I said before he said anything. I said, 'It's your
> own fault, you did it to yourself Mickey, you've only got yourself
> to blame'.

Merle suggests that health is not a priority for the clients. They take little notice of health advice, don't look after themselves and give greater priority to other concerns. From her own observations, Merle concludes that some clients have only themselves to blame when they get sick. In the face of these seemingly inexplicable and intractable behaviours, Merle feels thwarted.

Unlike clients in her previous health care experience, Merle's Family Care clients are not passive recipients of care within institutional settings. They live in the midst of obligations, responsibilities and priorities connected with both family and community relationships. This is particularly the case for grandmothers, who often care for the wellbeing of the whole family. Many of Merle's clients care for other family members. For example, in order to provide accommodation, they often jeopardise their rental agreements with the Government Housing Commission (GHC).

When Merle attempts to ascertain the extent of family support within client households, she also encounters mistrust. In a discussion on home visits, she shares this difficulty with her colleagues:

> I've been going to Phyllis for over a year and she won't even tell me who is staying there … It's a bit hard to, because sometimes they don't want to let you know who's living there with them, in case their agreement with the GHC is that they're the only person supposed to be there … Like Phyllis—even her son who died, he's on the GHC form and she's never had him taken off, although I've told her to tell them that he'd died.

Merle interprets Phyllis's reticence to share information as a concern with the GHC. However, her colleagues reveal that clients live in equal if not more fear of other government authorities:

> **June**: I think she's more protective about her kids because they're always in trouble with the law … and she's not eager to say whether she has them there or not … I would say that is the number one priority
> **Margie**: Yes it is—and Social Security.
> **June**: That's the other one.

Merle expects Phyllis to be honest, to confide in her and to heed her advice. She also believes Phyllis should be honest with the GHC. However, Phyllis has her own viewpoint. In particular, she has her own perspective on her relationship with Merle.

Not only do clients confide in Merle rarely, but in some instances they will not let her in the door. Some months later, she accepts the situation:

> Now for instance Topsy—every time she's got a full house, she never lets me in that front door … I know now that she doesn't want me to go in that house, so I don't make an issue of it. Before, I would have insisted, but now I just can't be bothered, because there's too many people in there that she shouldn't be having in there … the house is only for her and her daughter.

The case of Mimi and Fred

The following description of the relationship between Merle and her clients, Mimi and Fred, comes from observations and a series of interviews with Merle over almost a year. Mimi and Fred live in an outlying area, once agricultural but now part of the suburban sprawl. Mimi is fifty years old, diabetic and suffering from hypertension and anaemia. Fred is forty-eight, and suffers from diabetes with associated retinopathy, kidney disease, hypertension and gout. They live in the rear of a ground-level brick 1970s duplex.

Upon our arrival for a home visit, a young man of about seventeen sits on a front gatepost and checks us out. Merle approaches the door and asks if Mimi and Fred are at home. They are, and we go in and sit down in the living room.

Merle checks Fred's blood pressure, which is high (160/110), and his blood sugar level, which is low (2.1). He is almost blind and is on a disability pension. A letter on Fred's file indicates he has missed appointments at the Nephrology Department at the hospital. After Merle examines Fred, she begins talking to Mimi, who says she tries to keep her diabetes under control by using her own glucometer and checking her own blood sugar levels. Meanwhile, a relative of Fred arrives with a carton of beer, and he and Fred retire to the back garden.

Mimi's blood pressure is satisfactory (130/75), and her blood sugar level (7.0) more or less so. She tells Merle that she manages her own insulin injections and that she is careful with what she eats. She reports that she 'tries to feed her husband the right food'. At present, they have seven children living with them in the three-bedroom duplex, five of their daughter's children and two belonging to somebody else. After the visit, Merle tells me she cannot understand how people can live like that, with particular reference to 'the blokes going out the back to drink a carton of beer'.

Three weeks later, Merle tells me that in order to create some space to talk with Mimi she has organised a special appointment at the office. During the meeting, Mimi informs Merle that she has eight (not seven) children staying in the house. Merle says that they don't appear to go to school and that the twelve-year-old is asthmatic and goes off to discos and dances with her cousins without a puffer. Merle says Fred still has high blood pressure and drinks excessively, and that she told him he was in danger of having a stroke.

Merle reveals that the eighteen-year-old boy, who on our visit together surveyed us from the gatepost, used to sniff glue, now smokes marijuana, appears a bit slow and has never been assessed. The six-year-old and the nine-year-old both have bed-wetting problems. Merle thinks it would be a full-time job just to look after this family. She admits she gets frustrated: 'There are things to help people look after themselves, but nothing is happening'.

In Merle's view, Fred and Mimi's situation is 'typical' of that of many Aboriginal people. She wonders about the children's mother: 'Why have seven kids if you can't look after them? There's no excuse.' On another occasion, when she had organised some uninterrupted time at Mimi's home to sort out some of their problems, Mimi and Fred cut short her appointment by going out:

> You need to get the client sitting down with no distractions, but it's impossible … They were keen to get out and go to the park anyway—it's beautiful there. People wonder why they congregate in the park. When you see their living conditions, its obvious.

The following week Merle tells me that Mimi and Fred attended an appointment with Glenda, the social worker, concerning housing, and Glenda asked Merle to sit in. Apparently, Fred has now 'kicked [the eighteen-year-old boy] out of the house'. In the family, a thirteen- or fourteen-year-old boy and a twelve-year-old girl are both glue sniffers. The boy is in a detention centre and the girl is in trouble with the authorities. Merle reports that Mimi went to court, but one of the children did not show up.

Her clients do not always welcome Merle's assistance. She once rang Mimi and Fred in the late afternoon, concerning their medical appointment at the AHS the following morning. When she arrived at eight o'clock to pick them up, Fred said he was not coming and neither was Mimi, who had been up all night playing cards. Two months later, Merle reports:

> [Fred's] blood pressure is still up high, and then when you're talking to him, he's been out gambling all night—y'know, they've been to the casino all night. He might have got home at five o'clock in the morning, or just before I got there. I expect he probably drank while he was at the casino—he reckons he doesn't, but Mimi, when he's not there, she said, 'Yes, he does'. Actually, his blood sugar's not too bad, but his blood pressure's up to 170 … I keep telling him— I say to him, just for the shock effect, that he's going to have a heart attack in the casino … But he's good—he does win. I must admit, he's bought a video recorder for the kids, y'know. They can watch the video, and he's bought a stereo unit—all the records were there on Thursday when I went—plus he's got a big freezer.
>
> Then Mimi comes to me, and says, 'Oh, I've got to go and see Glenda, I've got a big light bill to pay'. So I said to Fred, 'Why didn't you go and pay your bill, instead of buying the freezer? Especially in this cold weather, you don't need a freezer'. And he said, 'Oh well', he said, 'We'll go and sell that, if we want some extra money, y'know'. So I said, 'Your freezer won't work if your power gets cut off, will it?' He said, 'Oh no, I s'pose it won't'… He's pretty good, y'know, he bought the freezer for her. But I was thinking at the time, though I didn't say it out aloud, but, why buy a freezer if [he] knew about the electricity bill?

Three months later, Merle reports more surprising news:

> Well, I think they've moved out! There's no furniture at their place—there's furniture under the carport, no furniture in the lounge. There was no curtains, so I could look in the window, and nothing in the kitchen as well … I didn't see them last week. I saw them down the street with my other clients—they were there down in the shopping centre, but I didn't stop the car 'cause I thought, y'know, they might be drunk or something. I've just rung the phone number for them, but there's no answer. I don't know where they've gone … I didn't see them the week before because they weren't there, I was told. There was a whole lot of people there playing cards, but someone came out before I had a chance even to get out the car, to say they weren't there—so I didn't want to push it. Whether they didn't want me to see them … I always get that impression—when someone comes out before you even have a chance to get out of the car. So that's what happened.

A further two weeks later, the whereabouts of Mimi and Fred arises in a Family Care meeting. Merle says that they left their house about six weeks previously and she has no idea where they are living. Ruby tells Merle that they rang and gave their address to Glenda, the social worker, who had forgotten to inform the healthworkers. Glenda has known where they are living the whole time. Merle responds, 'Now that makes me angry … they were seeing me and they never told me where they were shifting'.

Merle feels both unsupported by her clients and disrupted by their lifestyle and living context. At one stage she decides, 'I need to get the client sitting down with no distractions'. However, from overwhelming evidence she concludes that this apparently simple requirement is impossible. Children, visitors and her clients' own agendas consistently turn her plans upside-down. For Merle, the following facts stand out. Fred is already disabled and committed to a lifestyle that will cause more disability in the future. Financial management seems non-existent. Their unit is grossly overcrowded. The children do not go to school, are unwell, use drugs and are in trouble with the law. The range, depth and severity of this family's problems, and the synergistic mix of both clinical, social and psychosocial dis-ease, produces such a burden of need that Merle thinks it would provide sufficient work even if she had no other clients at all.

One way of understanding the disparate priorities of Merle and of her clients may be to reflect again on Merle's primary training and experience, which were within the biomedical context of a hospital. Her clients respond to biomedical issues, even life-threatening ones, as no more than everyday events, and for Merle this standpoint provokes deep frustration.

While client mistrust and priorities exasperate the healthworkers, Rose perceives that the wider social issues associated with poverty, inadequate housing and lack of education are equal sources of frustration. She considers these issues to be pivotal to the continued ill health of Aboriginal clients.

'It's the same problems'

According to Rose, the contribution of healthworkers is almost incidental to the endemic poverty among clients and Aboriginal families generally. 'It's the same problems', she says. The basic needs of elderly Aboriginal clients and their families, particularly their income and housing, are subject to frequent and serious disruption. Most subsist on minimal fixed incomes, such as disability or aged pensions. Unexpected financial demands often arise due to personal circumstances or disruption within the extended family. Financial constraints are evident from the numerous reports by healthworkers of clients needing monetary assistance, food packages, advocacy to negotiate bill-paying schedules and assistance with budgeting.

Rose attributes many of these problems to the clients' educational history, particularly exclusion from government schools. She despairs about the lack of general education of the elderly and its perpetuation among their grandchildren:

A lot of [clients] don't read and write—the grannies* don't even go to school. Kids of today don't do that—I don't know why. I think it's just that vicious circle again. Because their parents didn't have education, they don't see the importance of making their kids go to school.

Due to direct experience of social exclusion, cultural oppression and racism, many clients missed periods of schooling themselves, and have limited experience of mainstream social institutions, professions and public sector agencies. Consequently, some find it difficult to determine the status of service providers, as Monica, the care-aide, illustrates:

Because you work at AHS—when you go to see them and they've got something wrong with them, a cut or something wrong with them, they don't understand your position is just a care-aide. They think you're a doctor because you work for the Aboriginal Health Service, and that you can do these things like fix them up, give them stitches, or whatever. They expect you to do all this, just because you are associated with the AHS.

Conforming to the institutional regulations of the Government Housing Commission (GHC) frequently causes difficulties for clients. The problems range from overcrowding due to the arrival of homeless family members, elderly clients moving in with family to provide child-care support, and evictions, to the inadequacy of accommodation for chronically ill, frail-aged and disabled people. Rose describes what she means by satisfactory housing:

When I say housing, I mean having a nice home to live in, warm, with everyday comforts—where it's not freezing in winter and not cooking them in summer, not overcrowded. I'd say 90 per cent

---

*In this context 'grannies' denotes the grandchildren, not the grandparents.

of them, most of our clients [need alternative space] … and that has a large impact on their health and how they actually care for themselves.

Overcrowding is a problem, particularly where clients live with their extended family. Monica provides an example of interpersonal tensions affecting elderly clients:

At the moment, the situation here is [the clients'] daughter has left the son-in-law and they're in the middle of a divorce. Ken and Rona [the clients] at the moment feel uncomfortable living there because, y'know, he's only an in-law and it's his house. So tomorrow they've got an appointment with Glenda [the social worker]—so they can get Glenda to find accommodation for them. We're trying to get them into a place of their own without any family around—a lot of the time, the family interfere more.

Rose provides another example:

Take for instance one of the elderly clients at the moment. She's an asthmatic, she has a heart condition, she's living [in a shanty] on the river. Her health would improve greatly if she had a warm home to go to, to call home—a bed to sleep in. Maybe not even a bed—if she had a warm house … With the GHC, she doesn't pay her rent—that's a major factor, everybody has to pay rent. [The clients] need to understand they have to pay rent—they need to look at a way that their money can come straight out of their pension or whatever.

The healthworkers report that many clients receive large bills for rent arrears and repairs and, as a result, are in debt to the GHC. Liabilities for repairs often become a problem when clients provide refuge for other family members. Overcrowding results in extra wear and tear on houses, an outcome over which elderly clients have little control. However, as registered tenants they are liable for the costs.

Encouraging clients to 'take control'

Rose believes welfare dependency is one reason why clients do not pay their rent. She argues that historically legislated welfare dependence generated the 'hand-out system', and that it is because of the hand-out system that the elderly client living on the river will not pay rent:

> Basically, I think that all along it's been the hand-out system. The government's always been looking after [Aboriginal people], and all of a sudden the government's pulled away, and they're saying, 'No', and they've left these people floundering. They've had no education, no training, no nothing on how to take control of their own lives—and they've just walked away and said, 'Do it' … Even the younger kids, because of the way their parents were brought up, *that's* the way they have been brought up. So it's an ongoing vicious circle, where there'll be somebody there to look after you. It's always been done, so it'll continue to be done. But little do they know that it's *not being done*, that they have got to take control themselves. But that's a big thing—everybody knows they've got to pay rent, but they're thinking, 'Don't worry about it, somebody will be there to bail me out'.

This scenario applies equally to client relationships with other sections of the AHS and Family Care. In her leadership role, Rose attempts to implement practices, such as cleaning duties, that encourage clients and families to meet their own responsibilities:

> The cleaning stops at the client's bedroom if they've got anyone living in the house … If they've got a mob of people there, they're all using the bathroom, they're all using the toilet, and I think they can get off their [backsides] and clean—if they're adults … Alice [the previous Family Care cleaner] used to have the same problem with a family. They'd have big grown-up kids there, and they'd sit there and tell her what to do, and how to clean and what to clean.

Rose, like Rita and Josie, attempts to discriminate between essential services and inessential services that foster dependency. Nevertheless, within the broad ambit of Family Care's holistic approach, Rose senses some obligation to address other health needs in the client household:

> I don't expect you to run round in circles and make doctors appointments and all that. But I mean, just a routine blood pressure or something, coming in and making an appointment, that doesn't hurt anybody. And, with the way we're looking at holistic care, we've got to look at everybody—I mean we can't let somebody sit there dying beside you.

The healthworkers respond with concerns about the excessive time entailed in organising non-client appointments. By offering such a service, they fear family members will abuse it. Ruby provides an example:

> I just think once they know we'll refer them, they'll start asking us to refer them ... I did this for a client—she wanted to see Glenda, so I went and spoke to Glenda, made the appointment. Then I came back to ring the woman, and she wasn't home. So I had to go past on my way home and inform her the appointment was the next morning. She never showed up. Because I made the referral, I was Glenda's contact person, so Glenda chased me up.

After resisting Rose's initial suggestion, the healthworkers agree to provide information and contacts for other members of client households.

While Rose attempts to balance essential and inessential services in policy terms, healthworkers attempt to balance them in practice, as in this situation encountered by Merle:

> **Merle**: Like yesterday, just for instance, I was asked to take Mimi home. Halfway down Mission Street she said ... 'I've got a food voucher here for Coles—can you take me shopping?' So

you can't say no, you've got the car, the car belongs to AHS, y'know. So … I sat in the car and waited till she went shopping at Coles.

June: I'd ask if she needed it urgently … Do you need it now or can you get it tomorrow?

Ruby: They're gonna say yes.

Merle: The thing is they live far away at Peak Hill. I know they haven't got transport … And they've got to come in by bus.

June: They the ones way out there, eh? Oh, of course I would've done that.

Merle: Yeah, I think you would've done that June.

Ruby: Technically we could say, 'I finish at five. I'm sorry …'

Joan: I'd probably realise the sort of situation they'd be in. You do get to know each client and you know what sort of need …

Thus, in their evaluations of client need, healthworkers discriminate between dependency and genuine demand, based on their knowledge of the particular client and the context.

Rose understands that historical welfare dependency is systemic, and is often implicit in relationships between Aboriginal people and mainstream institutions:

The fact [is] that the hand-out system is there and they still go back to it—'That's what you are there for, to help us' … [Making services conditional] needs to be an overall thing. One organisation just couldn't do it, it would need to be a standard procedure right across, for Aboriginal people. It's a big issue. This is why a lot of people get into the problems they get into, with their housing and everything else—because they're helped out so much.

According to Rose, some families believe that a healthworker is responsible for 'looking after' a client, with 'looking after' implying constant vigilance, similar to a parent's supervision of a child. She offers an extreme example:

We were looking after Charlie's sister. She was one of these people that went around, got drunk and did her own thing, and it was very difficult to look after her. Anyway, on the weekend she got really drunk and got hit by a car, and it was sort of a fatal thing, and she ended up dying. Well, Nancy [Charlie's de facto] sort of blamed us, 'cause she reckons we were *looking after* her. '*Where were we?*', y'know, we should have been there, looking after her. That shouldn't have happened.

Rose's awareness of the hand-out system, her fear of perpetuating dependency and her concern with building people's capacity to take control themselves, underlie her standpoint on service provision. She advocates that the provision of services should be conditional on clients taking a more active role in meeting their own needs:

We don't really encourage them to be independent, because they know if they come to us we'll sort the problem out, which we do. They're not told, 'We'll sort out the problem this time—if you come again, you'll have to go to some education classes. We really need to work with you one on one, and look at the problem and see why it's happening all the time'. But it's just constant hand-out. For some families it may never work, but if you can get one out of twenty that becomes independent, that's a bonus … That's what we are trying to do with our elderly clients, making them take control of their own illnesses, for their own wellbeing.

She sees dependency and the hand-out system operating in other sections of the AHS, including the Medical Clinic and the Welfare section:

[The clients] don't really have to manage their own health, or to care for their own health … The doctors over the road, instead of telling them to take control of it, they're saying, 'Come back and see me tomorrow, come back and see me tomorrow, come back and see me tomorrow'… instead of saying, 'Go home. This is what

I want you to do, and I don't want to see you till next week' …
There's somebody there doing it for them, instead of them sort of
knowing that they have to take that control and do it themselves.

Rose perceives that hand-outs from other sections of the AHS
undermine Family Care's philosophy that clients should take control of
their own health, and Merle ridicules a suggestion by a social worker in
the Welfare section that healthworkers should clean clients' houses:

> I said to Glenda, 'Some of those houses are in the same condition
> every time we go'. [Glenda] said, 'Look at [names a client]. There's
> only one little thing that got her thrown out, and [the health-
> workers] could have prevented it by going out there and cleaning
> the house.' I said, 'I would never send any of the cleaners out there
> to clean that house. There's young people there, there's young
> women there that could clean the place out.'

While Family Care is committed to healing dependency, Rose
suggests that this is not so in other sections of the AHS, and that their
actions undermine the efforts of healthworkers to deliver services in an
appropriate manner. For Rose, dependency is a legacy from the past
that still lingers.

'Why am I doing it?'

Healthworkers find that the oppressive social context experienced by
Aboriginal people over generations continues to overwhelm clients and
their families. Legacies of exclusion and oppression are a major challenge to their effectiveness, and one consequence is a pervasive mistrust
of doctors, nurses and health institutions. Hence the considerable effort
healthworkers put into building close and trusting relationships with
clients, and the difficulty they often have in convincing clients to seek
or accept care.

Another historical legacy is a general lack of education, which
undermines efforts to instil health care messages and to encourage
the appropriate use of medication. Healthworkers report difficulties

'getting through' to clients in order to convince them to adhere to medication regimes for secondary prevention of chronic diseases. Clients are often misinformed about medications, either by unreliable sources or by short-term evaluations of drugs for curative rather than preventive qualities. All healthworkers are discouraged by the futility of endlessly repeating health messages that many clients ignore, and novices find this especially demoralising.

Inadequate housing and overcrowding, due to poverty, also take a toll on client health. Evictions cause clients even greater financial burdens, hardship and illness. Healthworkers attempt to balance the accommodation of client needs with encouragement for self-responsibility. However, because the hand-out system is part of the fabric of the institutional relationship between settler and Aboriginal Australians, and operative even in the AHS, their attempts to overcome dependency remain largely unsupported.

The experience of constantly confronting the past in the present leads healthworkers to despair that their task is 'endless' and almost pointless. They are often unable to assist clients either to benefit from health services or to take control of their own health. They perceive little progress in many clients whose health problems seem like a never-ending story.

BREAKDOWN IN FAMILY CARING

'They don't care like they used to'

June's experience demonstrates what she and her colleagues have discovered: that they can no longer count on the cultural tradition of families caring and taking responsibility for the elderly. The cultural ethic of 'share and care' is often distorted and, rather than younger adults caring for the elderly, the reverse is true. Whenever possible, June charges competent family members with the care of clients, and she encourages her colleagues to do likewise.

June herself is committed to family responsibilities. Like many Aboriginal people of her generation, June shared with many siblings, experienced bouts of illness in the family, removal from her family to a mission and an interrupted schooling. She was responsible for siblings at an early age and married early. June grew up in the rural wheat belt region. She left school at grade seven and never attended secondary school. Experiences of loss tinge her memories:

> That was a bit hard … in those days, we didn't have the opportunity to go to high school unless your parents had the money to pay your way. And then there was prejudice too. They didn't want Aboriginals in high schools getting the knowledge—and all that type of thing.

June developed an interest in health at eight or nine years of age, about the time she returned to her family after spending five years of her childhood in the same mission where her mother grew up. Her mother was a diabetic, and she taught June to inject insulin and to look after her needles:

> She was only in her late thirties, mid-thirties, and when I was about eight or nine she used to say, 'Come here and stand here, and I'll show you how to do my medicine. Now, I want you to draw it up through the needle, and this is where you put it.'

June's mother died at forty-two, and she stayed home to care for her father. Despite her hopes to become a nurse, June declined an offer of nursing training in another country town and took work as a domestic with a white family. She married when she was fifteen and remained in the rural wheat belt, where she raised her own seven children. Later, she moved to the city.

Now in her mid-fifties, June has status as a senior member of the Aboriginal community. She commenced work at the AHS in the early 1980s after completing in-house healthworker training. June has many years' experience in providing outreach services to Aboriginal families. In her work in the Family Care and Welfare sections and as the women's health officer, June has repeatedly confronted the breakdown of family caring relationships.

In a defining moment, June shares her deep concerns, and tells of how younger family members often take advantage of the elderly and compromise their wellbeing. Particularly distressing for June is the apparent unwillingness of young adults to take responsibility either for themselves or for others:

> You find a lot of elderly Aboriginal people that go to nursing homes … I remember one being in the Sunset Centre at one stage, and whatever pension money that was left over, that child would come, that daughter would come and take that extra money—that person would never have it. Y'know, that kind of thing. I don't know—the thing is, down through the ages of Aboriginal people we learned to share and care. But instead of teaching the kids, educating and saying, 'Now share and care, but you've got to learn to stand on your own two feet', y'know, 'Once you're married, that's your problem then', y'know what I mean. Or, 'When you get to a certain age, that's your problem', y'know, but still keep that love and nurture and caring for each other, still the same.

June's account reveals several central aspects of her experience of care of the elderly: 1) 'share and care' are traditional cultural values which have been handed down over the generations; 2) elderly clients are vulnerable to exploitation by young adults who misuse the teaching of 'share and care'; and 3) while maintaining 'share and care' as a cultural value, young adults need encouragement to take responsibility and stand on their own two feet. Both June and the other healthworkers despair at a situation where an elderly client's willingness to share and care is exploited by her own adult children, particularly when the client's wellbeing is compromised.

'They put their grandkids first'

The frail-aged and disabled clients serviced by Family Care are frequently grandparents who provide care for their grandchildren. They may care for two or three children at a time, who may range in age from infants to teenagers. The chronic illnesses from which most clients suffer make child-care arduous and further compromise their health.

Despite serious ill health, Nancy and Charlie care for their four grandchildren while the mother works. Josie reports that the grandchildren include a baby, whom they have cared for almost full-time since birth. The baby and an older boy live with Nancy and Charlie, and two other children often stay in their small home unit. Their father works on an oil rig off the coast, six weeks on and two weeks off. According to the healthworkers, even in his two weeks off, he leaves the children in the care of the grandmother.

Josie, who visits once a week, feels indignant about the whole situation. Heatedly, she describes a time when the mother did not see the baby at all for several weeks. She reports that following a mastectomy, Nancy is on chemotherapy, and has heart, liver and eye problems. As for Charlie, he recently had bypass surgery and is on multiple medications. Josie says Charlie is 'fed up' with driving the three children to and from school every day without even an offer of petrol money from their parents.

Fortunately, Nancy and Charlie receive significant support from Family Care. Besides Josie's weekly visits, the community development officer provides counselling sessions to Nancy, a care-aide provides respite and the cleaner services their two-bedroom Government Housing Commission unit weekly. The children, who are aged from thirteen downwards, are quite a handful:

> **Patty**: [The daughter said] that she would put the baby in full-time child-care, but Nancy felt that—because she was sick, and that the baby kept her mind occupied [she would continue to care for her]. But she didn't realise it was going to be full-time, even to her.
>
> **Merle**: Plus it's all the other kids as well.
>
> **Josie**: And that boy, he's really hyperactive isn't he?
>
> **Patty**: Yeah.

While the healthworkers recognise difficulties in the situation for Nancy, she is somewhat complicit with the arrangements. A suggestion that they approach the mother provokes intense discussion. Josie indicates that Nancy does not view the children as a problem or a burden:

Monica: The only other option is to call the mother of the children in—for the healthworker or for Family Care to call the mother in and talk to her about Nancy's health and let her know that what she's doing is just not helping Nancy at all.

Josie: But if we did that, would that feel like we were going over—going 'bout it over Nancy's head, y'know.

Monica: Well you'd think it shows that we care.

Josie: Yeah, but what I'm sayin' is that she might take offence to that … Every time I go there, I said, 'Look you got to learn to start saying no. You need time out for yourself.' I mean, there's only been once or twice where she, like, go Bingo, *and she takes all the kids with her*! Or she'll go to Johnny Cash and she's sayin', 'I'm gonna take the kids, or one of the grown up kids', or something. And I thought, 'Well gee, it's a night out for you and Charlie, so just go out and enjoy it'. 'If we weren't going to the casino afterwards, we would've taken one of the kids', that's her attitude. And I said, 'No! You gotta start thinking about yourselves.'

Later in the conversation, Rose declares that Nancy's behaviour is typical of most Aboriginal grandmothers:

The thing is, you'll find that's the general conception of most grandmothers of Aboriginal kids. I mean, they will put their grandkids first, and it's gonna take a hell of a lot to try and break that … And it doesn't really matter what age they are … it's part and parcel of most Aboriginal grandparents … I dunno, it's just being a grandparent … It is unhealthy … it's taking away the role too of the parent—'cause they're just thinking, 'Oh it is so much easier, because so and so will have the kids'. Y'know, they just palm them off, and they just breeze around and not have to worry.

Child-care provision emerges as a major issue affecting the well-being of many frail-aged grandparents. While the grandparents take on the caring role almost automatically, neither they nor the parents appear to realise the effects of child-care on their health. According to June, child-care can also frustrate the provision of health services:

It's frustrating—you can't do things without kids [being] there, y'know. And if you want to talk to [the clients] privately, about different things, then you can't do that. And if you've got to come into the doctor [with the clients], the kids are all in the car instead of going to school ... Nearly every second family you go to visit, they got them—some got little ones, some got, y'know, teenagers ... Just to give 'em a roof over their head ... they go and live with Nana and Pop ... Their own mum or dad over there [gestures], and they'll live with grandma and grand-dad ... [The children] couldn't be bothered with the parents see—frustrated ... so you get kids from nine, ten, eleven, twelve—grown up. That's what Kitty and Pete's got—they got kids from little knee-high kids to teenagers ... The parents will just shove 'em off on Nan and Pop.

June suggests that parents who are looking to free themselves from responsibility for their children, and children who are feeling neglected by their parents, all rely on grandparents. The burden imposed on Kitty and Pete upsets June.

Merle and I encounter the situation described by June when we visit Kitty and Pete. As we arrive, their daughters prepare to leave. Meanwhile, howls and screams come from a couple of grandchildren in the kitchen. As we enter the living room, three other children gather around, fighting and pestering each other. Shouting, laughing, crying and screaming fill the room. Merle attends to Pete:

Merle: How's your BP [blood pressure]?
Pete: Since these kids have been here it's probably gone up.

Outside in the car, Merle observes:

I don't think the kids realise how much pressure the grandparents are under. They probably don't even know they're sick. Those two should be in a nice little unit on their own … it's hard work having a conversation with kids screaming.

Later, the healthworkers explore why the grandparents take on the care of grandchildren. For some grandparents, it is apparently the only way to keep in touch with their family:

Ruby: But that's their role. A lot of grannies* are scared to give that up 'cause then they've got no value at all for their families.
June: Yeah.
Ruby: At least while they're lookin' after their kids, they're important to their family.
June: They [Kitty and Pete] are enrolled at the technical college—but they can't go because of the grannies [grandchildren].
Ruby: But then, their family doesn't come near them.
June: I dunno—well yeah—not just that one particular family.
Merle: Do you mean to say the family wouldn't come, just to see them, because—because they refused to have the kids? I mean, I refuse to have my grandkids, but they come and visit me.
Ruby: Yeah, but for some people it's a big problem.
June: Kitty and Pete have that problem.

Merle is disbelieving, but June confirms this situation and suggests that lack of trust towards day-care centres by some grandparents exacerbates it:

A lot of grandparents say, 'Well, if you can't look after them and you are going to put them in a day-care or whatever, I'll do it, regardless of how I am, and my condition'. Because a lot of them think of it this way: 'There's too much child abuse out there, regardless of what age they are—y'know. They're my grandkids, they're my kids—I'll take them, I'll look after them' … Don't give them to others. I'm like that with my kids.

---

*Here, 'grannies' refers to the grandparents.

Here, the contemporary legacy of the historical separation of Aboriginal children from their families surfaces within the discussion. June suggests that the fear of institutional abuse is never far from the minds of clients who are nominally members of the 'Stolen Generation'.

Merle gives a graphic example of a grandmother influenced by her own history. Because her own children were taken, she is unwilling to place her grandchildren in care, although she and they are homeless:

> When I went to Phyllis's … she wasn't there … Anyway, when I got round to Mimi's, she was there—she was saying her son got drunk and threw her out of her own home. She had the two little grandsons, his son's, with her … Phyllis looked awful—I s'pose you would if you were told to leave your house. The boys were there, but she said, 'No', she wouldn't go back, and she was worried about the little boys …
>
> Phyllis is reluctant to do anything [about putting her grandchildren into care] because her daughters were taken. She left them with these people, you see. She and her husband had to go and work—he worked for the railways and they got work wherever they could in the country. She left the two daughters with people, and when she came back they wouldn't let her see them.

Healthworkers indicate that the expectation that grandparents will care for grandchildren is cultural, and congruent with the tradition of share and care. Grandparents choose to look after their grandchildren, particularly when they perceive the children will be safer in their care than with potentially abusive institutional carers. Even more poignantly, grandparents undertake child-care duties in order to maintain close relationships with the rest of the extended family. For clients who have experienced separation from their families earlier in life, the threat of isolation is highly potent. Nevertheless, it seems that rarely are the detrimental health effects for elderly clients fully considered.

All this places healthworkers in a quandary. Mostly, they feel powerless to intervene in the complex web of family relationships, but they are very aware that care of children by elderly clients obscures awareness within families of their chronic illnesses. They also suggest it can result in parents failing to assume adequate responsibility for either their parents or their children.

'Old fellas are not respected'

Healthworkers perceive a general lack of care and respect for the elderly. They regularly encounter situations where the health and well-being of elderly clients appears to be of little concern to family members. Despite a traditional cultural value of respect for elders, Ruby perceives widespread exclusion of the elderly from their former central role in community life. Now, she suggests, the elderly have almost no status:

> **Ruby**: These old fellas have got nothin' really. If you think traditionally, they were the strong point of the community. Now, if they don't look after their kids or grandchildren, if they've got no role, they're choofed off to nursing homes, and they never get visited … They've got nothin'—they're not respected, families don't treat 'em nice.
>
> **Joan**: They don't care for each other like they used to.
>
> **Merle**: Well whose fault is that? Is it society's fault?
>
> **Ruby**: At least while they're looking after kids, they're staying [in the family] …
>
> **Joan**: They don't care for each other.
>
> **June**: I'd say it's the parents fault … lookin' after the grannies like they do.

It appears that a lack of care for the elderly is commonplace:

> **Ruby**: But some families are great to their oldies.
>
> **June**: Yeah.
>
> **Ruby**: There are a handful.
>
> **Joan**: Very few.
>
> **Ruby**: Most of them are abusive.
>
> **Merle**: You'd say the majority are.
>
> **Ruby**: I would say 90 per cent of the families don't give a damn about their oldies, but there are 10 per cent who do.

Not only do parents jeopardise the health of their own parents by placing grandchildren in their care, but healthworkers report that, in general, respect for elders is uncommon within client families. A case of extreme neglect causes Ruby deep disillusionment:

> Huh—here's a story. One old lady had a stroke, and laid on the lounge for three days, paralysed on one side, with a house full. There was at least thirty people in that house, and it wasn't till three days that a healthworker had gone in and picked up the lady that had the stroke, that the lady got treated.

June gives an example of adult children and other relatives taking food from an elderly client and leaving her dependent on welfare assistance:

> We had a couple of oldies—Welfare would do shopping for them. Pension day she'd be right, but the following week, before her pension again, she looking for food again, y'know. And because she was [at home by herself], she'd buy enough to just last her that one week … and the following week she'd be coming in, 'I need some food'. And Welfare asked her, 'Well, what happened last week?' … She had a daughter and son-in-law, and other relatives, who would come along and take [the food] too—poor old thing. An' that happens everywhere.

The healthworkers recount numerous instances of client neglect and deprivation of food and income at the hands of family members. With traditional relationships of care between the generations breaking down, they report cases where the actions of family members are tantamount to negligence. 'Specially when you've got a drinking family—and the majority of them are', says June.

Merle reports an instance where a client apparently has no expectation of care from his own family:

> He said he was thinking of another housing transfer and I said, 'Well how long have you been here?' And he said, 'Oh only a

couple of weeks—only moved in last week'. And I said, 'Well what's the matter?' And he said, 'Oh it's a long way to the shops'. And I said, 'Haven't you got anyone that can go shopping with you or take you shopping in the family?' And he said, 'Oh no, I don't think so'—and there's his son lying on the bed there asleep, in the lounge, where we were talking.

Sometimes, family members are concerned for their elderly relations solely in order to gain access to money. Indeed, in a discussion that focused on abuse of the elderly, June reports that grandparents will give money just to see their grandchildren:

> **Ruby**: A lot of old people are only in people's houses 'cause they collect their pension.
> **June**: Yeah.
> **Joan**: Yeah.
> **June**: They'll only look after them 'cause they got some money— 'Oh, pay day today' … Or if they living elsewhere, 'Well, we'll pop on down, it's mum or dad's pension today, they got some money'. And do you know what they do? Because they want the love and the care of that child to always be there—to see them, if that's the only time they can get seen, when their kids come and visit—they'll give them the money.

The healthworkers describe many instances where adult children financially exploit the tradition of share and care. One form of financial exploitation concerns carers' pensions, whereby the recipient of a carer's pension neglects their responsibilities. Ruby also observes how the provision of a carer's pension affects perceptions of caring responsibilities:

> [The relatives] will claim a carer's pension. They're not caring for that client, so then you go to someone else [in the family] and you say, 'Can you do this, this and this?' And they say, 'No. She [the other person] is getting the carer's pension, she should do it'.

Ruby suggests that some family members perceive a carer's pension as a wage for care-giving. The recipient is seen to be responsible for all care, thus relieving other family members of responsibility.

June reports on the case of an old man, and reveals how the exploitation of an elderly client fits into a wider pattern of abuse within a family:

The house is locked all day while [the couple who care for him] are at TAFE [College of Technical and Further Education]—and he's sitting out in the heat … [He is] uncle to her. She wants him to go into the Sunset Centre … but the de facto—the man, she's married to him now—her husband wants him there [so she can collect a carer's pension] … They lock the place up and leave him outside from 9 a.m. to 4 p.m. …

Before, he was alcoholic. He fell in the fire when he was drunk, and burnt all his legs—and he's had problems with other things. So the people I was seeing next door, they said, 'Can anything be done about the old fella there?' And I said, 'Well I gone to see the doctor, to get him to come out, to see if he can be put in the Sunset Centre, somewhere to be looked after while they're at [TAFE].'

Two or three times I was there. The house was just locked—he couldn't get in to have a feed during the day … The house was locked every day. He's out of the house … he's sitting out under a little palm tree, and the palm tree doesn't chuck much shade. Y'know we had the heat wave … when we had the 46 degree heat … the sun comes in at this angle, full strength on him. He gets up and sits in the chair where the palm tree is, and the palm tree doesn't throw anything at all—shade—if you're not sitting behind the trunk of it …

The niece … she's afraid of Max [her husband], 'cause Max is very abusive. Apparently he swore and carried on about it before. I said, 'I'm gonna have to come out here with Dr Rae. I don't care what he says, or what he does, because the old chap is my uncle as well'—and she, she's my cousin. And I said, 'I'm not going to let him sit out here, and Max abuse the hell out of you', 'cause he's not getting treated. She don't want to go to TAFE, but he's makin' her go along to TAFE because he [wants to be] with her every day. He don't want her home, 'cause he's afraid others will come back and forth.

Here, June perceives the old man's mistreatment originates with the husband, who also abuses his wife. Because the husband is jealous and constantly requires his wife to stay with him, she is unable to remain at home to care for the old man despite receiving a carer's pension.

Not only is there a lack of care for the elderly by their own off-spring, but healthworkers confirm instances of grandchildren abusing their grandparents:

Monica: But there's some of these grannies [grandchildren] that physically rough their grannies up to get this money, y'know. It's got to the stage now where they just give in and give it to them, because they're sick of getting punched around or pushed around ... by little kids.

Rose: These are little kids, nine, ten and eleven years old.

June: You can try and argue with them, but they don't respond to anything.

When confronted by the abusive treatment of clients, healthwork-ers report that they often feel compromised and frightened:

Rose: Because it's not only just the financial abuse. I mean, we've got a couple of clients in the nine years that I've been here that we know have been getting the physical abuse. You know some-thing's been ... so they are being physically abused, but because they're not going to talk to us or won't dare talk to us, you've just got to walk away—because you can't do anything. I mean you can't say to the family, 'Oh well what happened?' and they say, 'Oh I just fell over', knowing that she can't move out of the chair on her own anyway. So you've just got to face that.

Merle: With that too, they might tell you, but you can go back the next day and they'll deny it … It's not that we don't want to get involved with them, we're frightened … It's like Marlene, you know the black eyes, I don't know how many black eyes she's had … she always tells you the door, she ran into the door.

Incidents of alcohol-related violence, physical, financial and emotional abuse of clients discourage and frighten healthworkers. They have few professional guidelines and little organisational support. Rose thinks the extent of client abuse requires action:

We need to be able to do something because there's so much of it out there, see … 'Cause I mean there's emotional abuse, there's financial abuse … physical, sexual—I mean it's all there and it's all happening … We've got a couple of clients on our programme that have been sexually abused, we've got so many that are financially abused, we've got so many that's even emotionally abused and the ones that, I mean there's physical ones out there too, but they're not talking about it. And you know that it's happening and [health]workers are going into their homes on a regular basis.

Healthworkers perceive that many adult children compromise the health of chronically ill clients. Client provision of child-care and dependence of adult children both undermine client health and well-being. Often dependency becomes abusive. Adult children exploit their elderly parents to secure carers' pensions or rob them of their pension money or food. Healthworkers also encounter instances of physical, emotional and sexual abuse, but find that many clients are unwilling to take further action. In brief, the healthworkers perceive little evidence of the cultural tradition of 'share and care', nor of respect for elders. Rather, they confront widespread cases of exploitation, abuse and neglect.

Constrained by a code of silence

When confronting the abuse of their clients, healthworkers also express concerns about their own safety. Rita describes how she felt too scared to intervene on behalf of the old man locked out of his house (described in the previous section):

> **Rita**: See, I'm not going to get involved with this. It's dangerous. Because [her] husband is a very violent man, and I think it's dangerous for all of us. June's his niece—well, that might be a bit different, [he] might be different towards her. Because I mean I'm a stranger and I feel like that it's not my place to go and pick [the old man] up and take him to the Sunset Centre—because the family don't want him to go, y'know what I mean?
>
> **Ruby**: It's easy to make a policy when you're sitting in an office. But if you're the healthworker going to see the client, they know where the complaint's coming from.

While Rita recognises that any intervention could endanger her own safety, Ruby perceives that their regular consultation with clients readily identifies healthworkers as informers, and puts them in danger of revenge, or 'payback'. Nevertheless, Rose suggests that healthworkers have a duty of care when faced with elder abuse and that, by ignoring it, they become complicit:

> **Rose**: We're just as much to blame as the family if we are going to stand by, and go in every day and every week watching this and knowing it's happening and then walking away and saying, 'Oh, that's nothing to do with me'. Because it is something to do with us. This is where healthworkers are involved in the client, and we're falling down in that client's care because we just don't want to get involved with the family.
>
> **Merle**: It's not that we don't want to get involved with them— we're frightened.

According to Rose, a code of silence surrounding family abuse entangles healthworkers, whom she believes have a professional responsibility to act. Nevertheless, Merle also fears becoming involved. The healthworkers perceive that the code of silence about abuse and the history of clients are closely linked:

> **June**: When you look at all of our people there, the majority of them who we see, the one's we see like out there … they're all the Stolen Generation, y'know the stolen children, y'know what I'm sayin'. The majority of them won't bring up their pain because they were strapped on the knuckles—'*Shut up!*', '*Sit!*', '*You don't do … !*' And they've had it, they've had it all, yeah— and they're sort of survivors from it, and they're not going to come out and tell …
>
> **Ruby**: Most of them of 'em 've had shit happen to them all their lives. What's one more little bit of shit.
>
> **Rose**: Yeah, and they've coped with it all.

It is through this code of silence that societal oppression becomes inter-nalised within Aboriginal families.

Being part of the community themselves, healthworkers also fear for the safety of their kin. Monica says that if healthworkers intervene, a client's whole family is likely to become embroiled:

> The biggest problem with this, or with us, is in dealing with fam-ily problems. It becomes a bigger issue with that family … where the whole family becomes involved and they get physical, verbally abusive and start making threats, and then it comes to the point where you're afraid of your own life—especially like for health-workers. Like if Christine was coming and saying that Mrs X was being raped by her carer, and we do something, then that carer's family is going to become involved and then start threatening Christine or making up stories, y'know.

Monica describes the verbal abuse suffered by her own daughter at school, and how it extends beyond the school playground to the public arena, where she has been abused by another child's mother and aunties. In the healthworkers' experience, threats to one person become the basis of tension between families.

I asked the healthworkers whether there was a lot of fear in the community:

> **Christine**: I live in fear every day. I'll go home, and the first thing on my brain is, 'I hope that so and so's not drunk when I walk in the front door'—and I walk through the door. And as soon as I walk up he turns me inside out—and I do that *every day*, yeah. And you can just imagine what these other poor fellas are going through—yeah. Well, I can see I'll have to have him get out of the house for our old age.
>
> **Monica**: But with some Aboriginal families, abuse has been going on for years … That is one of our biggest problems we're gonna have I reckon—is the family and conflict.

The healthworkers practice within a community context in which injurious relationships are common. They encounter abusive relationships not only in client families, but sometimes in their own. A code of silence often surrounds such situations, and although they aspire to address abuse, they too become complicit with the silence. One reason why they prefer not to act is the lack of clear practice guidelines and organisational support. Another is fear for their own safety and that of their family.

'Getting young people to stand on their own two feet'

June believes that the central factor in cases of abuse is the dependency of young adults. In her work with families, she observes that many young adults are dependent on their parents and seem unwilling to take responsibility either for themselves or for their own dependents. To break this dependency, she sees a need for improved parenting skills and greater encouragement for young people 'to stand on their own two feet'. However, on the basis of their own experiences, her colleagues remain sceptical of the possibilities of transferring specific child-raising skills to young Aboriginal parents:

> **June**: A lot of them aren't strict enough in their own home, with their kids. If [they say], 'Oh mum, I'm sick today'—y'know,

put on act, 'I'm sick today'—'OK' (very gentle hushed voice) … Where they should get the kids off—'C'mon now' (briskly), 'It's your turn now, you gotta go to school. If you don't do this … you're not going to get this type of job when you get older, you won't have a certificate to get into this', or whatever … sit down and talk to your kids. But there's no communication, there's no communication. Kids are out on the street running around, seven- and eight-year-olds, 'cause mum and dad …

Ruby: Are drinking.

June: Or sittin' around playing cards, or they're at the casino.

Ruby: Drinkin', druggin'.

June: Or friends are around drinkin' y'know, that type of thing.

Merle: Like these kids grow up thinking drinking, that's normal.

June: Y'know what the kids think, in their lives when they get older? These mob didn't look after me when I was this age, so why should I worry about them. 'F— them, they get no-way', y'know that's how it is, some of them. That's how it is out there. Traditional times it was different—a lot, lot different.

June feels that communication with both children and young adults is critical. She advocates communication that asserts leadership and imposes conditions and limits on care:

A lot of [young parents], most of them need guidance … They get their dole—or supporting parent's pension, the first thing they do is go and buy their kid a toy … You can't do that, afford that every pay! 'That's for your birthday' or 'That's for Christmas' or a special occasion, 'if you're good'. That's bribing a child, but I usually do that [laughs]. I'd say, 'If we have to get this, and we get that, then we won't have that, or this, for next feed'—or whatever, y'know.

She believes it important for parents to maintain close communication with their young children and to set conditions on their demands early in life. She also thinks it important to teach parents to maintain a firm commitment to consistency—for instance, to ensure regular attendance at school. Concerning young adults, June advocates the need to place limits or conditions on parental generosity. She uses her experience with her own adult children as an example:

> Because I'd say to them, 'Rightio, I'm lending, loaning you this. Next week, when I want it back, I want you to come and give it to me in full, not half.' So they'd come and give it to me.

June highlights the conversational mode, which can be used to encourage self-responsibility while at the same time maintaining a loving relationship:

> Saying, 'Now share and care, but you've got to learn to stand on your own two feet', y'know. 'Once you're married, that's your problem then', y'know what I mean. Or, 'When you get to a certain age, that's your problem', y'know, but still keep that love and nurture and caring for each other, still the same.

According to June, negotiating with and setting conditions on support for young adults ensures that such support and care is not taken for granted or assumed as a right. She considers that this style of communication can work for healthworkers, particularly when charging family members with the caring role.

Ruby describes a situation that arose while transporting a client, her children and some companions. When she accommodated the adults' request to stop so they could go shopping, she was left with the care of the children. June is adamant she would not provide such a service: 'I would have said, "No" ... You've got to put a stop somewhere along the line, because if that's gonna happen, we're gonna have it all the time.' June strongly advocates drawing a line or setting limits on requests for assistance from both clients and their relatives. She insists that people learn to stand on their own two feet:

> **Ruby**: Then—these four little starving kids ...
> **Joan**: They're not that completely useless or hopeless—I'm sorry.
> **June**: They're really not. They depend on us, they're dependent and they've got to learn not to depend, know what I mean ...

If we keep doing it, and doing it, and doing it, they gonna depend on that role.

Joan reports an occasion where she forgot to organise transport for a client. A family member was at home with a car but neglected to assist, a situation that Joan accepted. June's response suggests indignation. She reports that when faced with a similar situation herself, she charged the daughter with the care of the mother:

> I turned to the daughter-in-law and I said, 'Look, *you're home—what are you doing*? Your mother-in-law needs to get to the doctor, straight away' … And she lives way out woop woop—up there. So what happened? She said, 'I'm going back into work shortly', and I said, 'Well look, don't go. You take [the client] to the doctor, stay with her, and then you take her home.' And she done that …
>
> I could've taken her myself, but I thought, here they are, she's without medication, and how many days she been without? And she's way out there by herself, and she's got two able-bodied persons, her son and her daughter-in-law, that was trotting back and forward to work, not sorting out mum—'Have you got all your medication?', whatever, y'know that type of thing …
>
> I think if children live in the home with them, right, surely if the parents can provide a roof over their head they can help out a fair amount. Surely they can do that.

While Joan agrees with the idea of getting people to stand on their own two feet, June is prepared to act on it. In this case, she encourages the daughter-in-law to take on the care of her mother-in-law, and challenges the underlying assumption that it is primarily the healthworker's role to look after the health of the client.

Crucial to the separate approaches of June and Joan are their differing backgrounds in relation to status and training. June, a senior member of the Aboriginal community with a depth of experience and training as a healthworker, deals both skilfully and successfully with the situation. In contrast Joan, a younger care-aide with little experience and minimal training, is unable to issue a challenge.

Merle also has difficulty asking a family member to look after one of her clients. She is a trained healthworker, but she is less experienced than June and not from the local community:

> **Merle**: Like I couldn't say to her that her husband had head lice on his arms … Every time I go there he's got them on his arms … I dunno, I might be the only one that sees them.
>
> **Joan**: And you couldn't tell her?
>
> **Merle**: No, but I told one of the grand-daughters. I said, 'I'm gonna give you stuff for his arms, he's got head lice on his arms'. But they hadn't done anything about it y'know, so I brought some stuff out. But then a couple of weeks later he still had the scratching … and the other day I was sitting there, and I was flicking them off his arm.

Merle indicates that the client's wife intimidates her, and that is why she resorts to informing a younger family member of the client's need.

Nevertheless, June suggests that as they become familiar with family members, healthworkers can ascertain their potential as carers:

> Quite often you can tell when a person's responsible and you can talk sense to them … and quite often there's a few you can't talk to either, y'know what I mean … You can assess them by seeing their actions, knowing who they are, what they do.

One strategy for directly addressing the issue of dependency on healthworkers is to charge family members with the care of their elderly. June demonstrates how communication that asserts leadership and sets limits can engage family members with the carer role. This approach actively challenges the idea that the healthworker is primarily responsible for the care of elderly clients.

THE COMMUNITY CONTEXT

A fraught healing space

Visiting clients in their homes is a large component of the healthworkers' practice. During this study, I accompanied them on home visits to about one-third of their clients. These visits varied in duration and location, and in terms of the number of family members present. Usually, healthworkers conferred with clients alone, or together with one or two family members. Sometimes an extended family group was present. While some clients were bedridden, most were active despite their chronic illnesses.

Generally, the format of a home visit was as follows. The client invited the healthworker inside, and the healthworker made initial enquiries about their health and recent activities. In most instances the conversation extended to the wellbeing of the client's immediate family members. The client usually sat at the kitchen table or in a convenient chair to enable the healthworker to take their blood pressure and, if necessary, their blood sugar level. When clients showed an elevated blood sugar level, the healthworker usually asked when they had last eaten, whether they had been taking their tablets or insulin, and about their level of exercise. Often the healthworker advocated the benefits of exercise and a healthy diet. Likewise, when clients displayed a high blood pressure reading, the healthworker usually investigated their medication schedule and stress levels.

After recording blood pressure and blood sugar levels in her diary, the healthworker routinely inquired further about the client's medications, about any alterations in the specific medicine or dose, and whether the client had sufficient medication until the next visit. They usually checked to see if any other medical supplies were required, such as Vicks, Ventolin, Betadine, salves for skin irritations, gauze pads or analgesics, and these were supplied without charge.

When clients reported particular ailments, the healthworker either advised them directly or arranged an appointment with a doctor. Where a client advised that they had a future appointment with a specialist, the healthworker normally offered to accompany them or to arrange the transport.

In most of the home visits, I observed a paramedical or narrow clinical approach. The average length of the visits I observed was eighteen minutes, and they ranged from five to forty minutes. However, I doubt that this was typical, as I sensed that my presence prevented healthworkers from engaging clients in depth.

Home visits sometimes included attendance at medical appointments with clients. Twice I accompanied a healthworker and client to outside (non-AHS) consultations, one at a hospital and one with a local general practitioner. From leaving the client's home until we returned, the hospital consultation took four hours and the doctor's consultation one hour.

According to the daily roster sheets, on average the Family Care healthworkers made between five and six home visits per day. Those in the Chronic Care programme averaged eight visits. Over six months, client files indicated that on one-third of home visits, clients were absent. My own observations matched this data: healthworkers spent almost half their time in the office, where they followed up client needs, attended to administrative tasks and debriefed with each other.

While I was able to observe healthworker activities with clients in their homes, I gained no more than a snapshot of the client's circumstances and I lacked a meaningful temporal and social context for these interactions. In contrast, the healthworker was normally aware of the client's history and their immediate social context, and sometimes shared this knowledge with me before we arrived, as in these three examples:

> The boyfriend's on metho, the niece died, she has a nephew in gaol, her grand-daughter's on kidney dialysis and her sister recently died.

> We're trying to get them into a place of their own without any family around—a lot of the time the family interfere more.

> [The son's partner] doesn't want [his children]. She's been in gaol and when she comes out she's going up north. This woman [the father is] with ... she's got six children she can't look after—someone else has got them. [The client's] got an old gentleman friend ... The son was standing over the old bloke and bashing him up and telling him not to come around ... threatening and wanting to take money off him to buy drink.

Knowledge of the myriad health and social issues that affected the lives of the clients informed the visit for the healthworker.

Home visits in the community evoked within me a range of responses. For instance, the extreme nature of Daisy's circumstances (see Chapter 4) was striking. Not only was she obviously very ill, being bed-ridden, on home dialysis for renal failure and recovering from a heart attack, but she suffered continuous pain from gangrenous toes and bedsores. Equally distressing was the fact that her bed was in the front living room of an already overcrowded house. The visit prompted the following journal note:

> Immediately, experiences in remote northern communities of Aboriginal Australia come to life in my memory—the different concepts of living space across cultures—however here we are in a modern city—I am confronted by the arising of my own needs— my personal concept of a healing space—and the space this old lady is existing within does not meet it—kids running amok, people coming and going, noise, emotional outbursts, litter, flies circling—it feels so harsh to me—it fills me with feelings of unknowing, not having a handle on what I am experiencing—a sense that this is way out of my reach and a desire to bring some control into the situation—I become aware how my recent meet-ings with Aboriginal Australia have been cushioned by comfort-able offices and meeting spaces.

Daisy's circumstances provoked an immediate heightened awareness of my own privileged existence and my immunity from the overcrowding and poverty that many Aboriginal people experience daily. On further reflection, my patronising reference to 'the different concepts of living space across cultures' is significant. Daisy had few choices about her living situation, as poverty limited her options.

A client of Merle also lived in an overcrowded house:

> We walk in and the old man is sitting in the lounge room with his son and daughter-in-law—we go in and the healthworker speaks

loudly to the partially deaf old man to introduce herself—his son sits on a straight-backed wooden chair in the lounge room leaving his half-full bottle of beer sitting on the floor underneath his chair untouched—pictures of family, some works of Aboriginal art and sporting trophies cover the walls—two nephews featuring in the photos in their football gear turn out to be wearing guernseys of a team from within gaol—the healthworker takes the old man's BSL and BP—we leave—after seeing the client we talk about the messy state of the house and the rubbish on the floor.

Again, the circumstances are impoverished, and they include chronic illness, unemployment, overcrowding, poor quality housing and imprisonment of family members. As family members watched proceedings, Merle attended the client. Because he was deaf, Merle had to shout. All present were privy to the consultation. After taking his blood pressure and blood sugar level, the family members requested check-ups, which the healthworker provided. The social context of the visit made it almost impossible for the healthworker to engage in a sustained dialogue with the client.

Communication with clients was often disrupted by grandchildren. During a home visit with Merle, the consultation was dominated by children coming and going from the living room:

Merle goes to the door and announces herself—the couple invite her in and we enter a front room with vinyl floors, an old couch and a couple of straight-backed chairs—there are two dressers covered in trophies and family photographs—a boxing trophy dominates one of the dressers—there's a couple of photos of young men in prison garb. It is the middle of school holidays and the couple's grandchildren are there—they tell us they have sixteen altogether—five of them are present while we are there—the first fifteen minutes of the visit there is a background of howling and screaming children … Merle arranges to visit them on a Wednesday afternoon, after 2 p.m. when there will be no grandchildren present.

The noise and confusion generated by the children, and the apparent acceptance of it by the clients, were astonishing. No one seemed at all concerned. Again, a preference for a quiet and private consultation arose in my mind.

Healthworkers sometimes met with clients alone, which allowed them to converse more easily:

> The healthworker takes the client's blood sugar level and finds that it is fourteen … The healthworker tells her a good twenty-minute walk will bring it down. The client says she will go for a walk around the yard. The healthworker takes her blood pressure which is in the normal range. The healthworker tells the client that her blood sugar level is a problem and she needs to watch her diet. The healthworkers talks to her about food preparation and offers to get her the diabetic cook book.

In essence, it was apparent that poverty, unemployment, over-crowding and stress marked the lives of many clients. The circumstances within which chronically ill people were attempting to manage illnesses were extremely trying, both for the clients and for the healthworkers.

The normality of dis-ease

Pervasive chronic illnesses were often a part of the healthworkers' own family lives, and they exhibited a sense of inevitability about persistent illness, sickness and death. This was particularly evident when measuring clinical indicators and then giving advice about disease management. Their persistent exposure to uncontrolled chronic disease seemed to influence their advice to patients, which often differed from that of other health professionals.

This variance was particularly evident with diabetes. Client files indicated that 53 per cent of the Family Care clients were diabetic. A frequent intervention by healthworkers for clients with Type 2 diabetes was advice about maintaining medication schedules, the benefit of exercise and the necessity to monitor diet. However, while according to the doctors and the nurses, the 'normal' blood sugar level was 4–8 mmol, some healthworkers reported that they considered readings of up to 11 or 12 as 'normal'. According to one healthworker:

> You allow for that little bit extra. It's when you have got 16s and 20s it's a problem. Some people are 24, and these blackfellas just walk around with it. Other people couldn't take it, they can take it—at about 14 it worries me.

Another healthworker, when asked what she considered a reasonable blood sugar level, replied:

> Between about 4 and 12-ish—say 4 and 11—but if they go over a little bit [it's OK]. Not only that, but I look at their past sugar levels to see what area or number they're at, that's sort of normal.

Rather than using the accepted biomedical norm for blood sugar level, it appeared that some healthworkers used a norm averaged from the population they serviced. Because readings were consistently high among their clients, some healthworkers routinely accepted high readings as 'normal'. This may partly explain a perception by the Family Care field nurses and some doctors (see Chapter 3) that healthworkers did not appear to follow up persistently high readings. Within a context of endemic Type 2 diabetes, reported to affect 25 per cent of the population serviced by the AHS,[2] healthworkers seemed to have shifted the parameters of 'normal' readings.

The close familiarity of healthworkers with the problems of their clients was evident in the fact that most, or at least some of their kin, lived in similar social conditions and experienced similar health concerns. For instance, during this study one healthworker arrived at work after police raided her house, searching for drugs that were alleged to be in her son's possession. She described the contempt with which police had treated her person and home; how they had 'kicked her things round with their feet, pulled everything out of her cupboards and just *shoved* it all back'. Another healthworker took extended leave to help her son in his attempt to overcome an amphetamine addiction and avoid gaol on related charges of stealing. Two of the healthworkers lived in abusive relationships, one with an alcoholic and the other with a heroin user. One healthworker described her job as dealing with 'everyday problems, y'know, problems that I deal with myself in my own life':

> Sometimes I walk out of their places really drained, because I've got problems of my own. You've got to leave them at home and do your work—husbands being drunk and drug addicts. And, y'know, beating them up, no food. Things like that happen everyday—kids going to court and stuff like that …

Healthworkers were sometimes clearly unable to commit fully to their work due to all-consuming personal or family problems, and sometimes the team leader challenged them about their performance. One healthworker, who was subject to such a challenge, reported:

> There's times when I've been slack and there's other times when I'll be really committed. Everyone goes through stages … [when I'm slack] I won't keep up with my bookwork or files, or I won't follow up things in general. Like I'm not doing my work right and I know that. But when you've got other things as well, that you've got in your personal life, and things interfering all the time …

Commitment to their work varied between the healthworkers, particularly in the provision of comprehensive, holistic home visits. Sometimes the variation in home visits appeared to result from the immediate context of the client or from conflicting professional or personal demands on the healthworker, but there were also differences in the commitment of healthworkers—as Karen, the field nurse, observed:

> There's a lot of different personalities between the healthworkers here, so the role is quite different amongst all of them. And their expertise, depending on what expertise they have, will depend on what knowledge they can pass on to a client.

Ruby, however, felt that personal concerns should not interfere with the work:

> Good healthworkers set priorities—they don't let personal and family commitments get in the way, they want to change things. They are the ones who don't stay a long time. They get *that* sick of it, they move on or burn out.

In brief, the circumstances of the clients often reflected difficulties the healthworkers confronted in their own lives, and sometimes the healthworker's own problems were so pressing that they diminished their capacity to perform their duties.

OUTCOMES OF EXCLUSION AND OPPRESSION

Three central dilemmas mark the experience of healthworkers: the scope of their practice, the response of the client, and the extent of caring and support within client families. In general terms, the challenges created by the broad scope of their practice often place the healthworkers under pressure. Their clients' dispirited responses dishearten them, while mistreatment of the elderly by family members both saddens and frightens them. A significant thread connecting these dilemmas is poverty. The legacy of the poverty includes persistent financial problems, inadequate housing, recurrent illness, social alienation, mistrust and dependency. The healthworkers associate these contemporary social issues with intergenerational patterns of social exclusion, cultural oppression and racism.

The healthworkers base their service provision on their conception of a holistic practice. That practice encompasses a wide range of complex needs relating to clinical, environmental, social and psychosocial wellbeing. Pivotal to it is their role as 'middleman', offering transport, advocacy and emotional support to clients unsure and mistrustful in their dealings with mainstream service providers. In some instances, the healthworkers admit to feeling overwhelmed by the unconstrained breadth of their practice. Sometimes, the complex and time-consuming needs of one client inhibit their ability to service other clients. Persistent social needs often take priority over clinical concerns, to such an extent that healthworkers with basic clinical training even question their designation as a *health* worker.

Conflicts occurs between healthworker agendas and client priorities. Within their holistic role is the expectation that the healthworkers will engage clients in health education and initiate behavioural changes concerning exercise and diet. However, clients are often uninterested, unwilling or incapable of engaging. Frequently, the presence of family members, the client's own personal plans, or competing demands on the healthworker determine events during home visits—making in-depth dialogue with the client about health impossible and only narrow biomedical monitoring feasible.

A holistic practice exposes the healthworkers to unpredictable demands. Sometimes they feel their compliance with client demands fosters dependency. Demand comes not only from clients, but also from other health professionals who, with scant regard for their existing commitments, co-opt healthworkers' assistance. Subject to multiple demands, one healthworker exclaimed, 'There is not enough of you'.

The dispirited response of clients also poses a dilemma. In large measure, the healthworkers attribute this response to lack of education, lack of self-confidence and mistrust due to experiences of social exclusion, cultural oppression and racism. The healthworkers find that many clients transfer onto them a deep-seated mistrust of health professionals and health institutions. Consequently, they spend considerable effort building close and trusting relationships with clients based on their own Aboriginality. They perceive that their informal relationships and frequent visits enable them to continuously monitor health, educate clients, provide support, and encourage clients to 'take control'.

Nevertheless, the healthworkers often have difficulty 'getting through' and gaining a positive response from clients. They attribute negative responses—which include judging medications prescribed for secondary prevention on their curative qualities, self-testing the efficacy of medications over short periods, accepting anecdotal evidence about drugs and their side effects and blaming medications for unrelated symptoms—to client mistrust and lack of education. The healthworkers also report difficulty in instilling messages about healthy behaviours. While they suggest that previous experiences of social exclusion affect client responses, they also indicate that continuing social problems relating to poverty and marginalisation undermine client priorities.

Another systemic factor undermining client health is the lack of self-confidence among clients, which according to the healthworkers is a legacy of legislated welfare dependency or the 'hand-out system'. The healthworkers claim that clients believe they will be 'looked after' by government welfare agencies and other social service providers. They attempt to overcome this dependency by discriminating between essential and inessential needs, based on their local knowledge. However, the operation of the 'hand-out system' in mainstream social service agencies and within other sections of their own agency undermines their attempts to encourage clients to take control of their own health.

The response of family members creates yet another dilemma for the healthworkers. Within families, the healthworkers find that traditional cultural values, such as 'share and care' and 'respect for elders', may no longer operate. Often they find chronically ill clients caring for grandchildren, to the detriment of their own health. While traditional cultural expectations of grandmothers prompt such efforts, they sometimes result from threats of isolation from the family or fears about the safety of children in child-care.

Clients may be subjected to fear and coercion within their own families and may also suffer from neglect, lack of respect and inadequate care. The healthworkers report elderly clients left destitute after providing food, money and shelter to their adult children. Where alcohol abuse is a problem, the healthworkers are unable to involve other family members in client care, and dependency and exploitation of elders may extend to financial, emotional, physical and sexual abuse. As they are privy to family secrets, a code of silence ensnares the healthworkers. Fear for self and their own kin precludes intervention. The unwillingness of clients to publicly disclose such occurrences also dissuades the healthworkers from further action. Only one healthworker in the study demonstrated the capacity to charge family members with the necessary care of their elderly; the others, who had less community status, found it more difficult. In essence, the practice of these outreach healthworkers is characterised by the uncertainty, disruption and chaos prevalent within Aboriginal family and community life.

In the face of these myriad dilemmas, on what basis do these healthworkers undertake their work? The healthworkers engage their work with a particular understanding of what constitutes Family Care healthworker practice.

A unique client-centred holistic practitioner

The healthworkers conceive a Family Care healthworker to embody Indigenous values, Indigenous understandings of the contextual determinants of client health, a particular set of objectives to enhance client wellbeing, and a matching set of culturally appropriate practices. They see their practice as being culturally appropriate, client-centred and holistic.

Thus they operate with deference to a variety of realities common to the lives of their Aboriginal clients. The pervasive social disruption within client lives, the unpredictable character of home visits and the shifting circumstances of many clients require healthworkers to be open, flexible and client-centred. Specific psychosocial legacies, such as client dependency, demand cultural understandings, appropriate judgement and specific negotiating skills. The healthworker establishes an Aboriginal style of relationship to assuage client mistrust of health professionals, to facilitate access to the necessary care and to maintain health-enhancing behaviours.

Their holistic practice encompasses basic clinical practices directed towards maintaining and monitoring the physical wellbeing of clients, social advocacy practices centred on alleviating issues linked to poverty, educational practices related to prevention, and emotional support practices linked to cultural and family health. While clinical practices focus on the physical health of clients, healthworkers direct social, educational and support practices towards change, either within the client or within their circumstances. The work draws on knowledge of both clients and their family relationships.

While a holistic practice provides a sufficiently broad scope to deal with client demand, healthworkers are sometimes overwhelmed by the magnitude of this demand. How other employees in the health service perceive the practice of healthworkers is the focus of the next chapter.

Working Alongside Healthworkers

The previous chapter alluded to underlying tensions between Aboriginal healthworkers and other health professionals, including doctors, social workers and nurses. Some of these tensions concern respect for the professional status and practice loads of healthworkers, the demarcation of practice boundaries, service delivery protocols, the prevention of client over-servicing and the perpetuation of historical patterns of dependency. Having looked at how healthworkers understand the nature of their practice, what are the perceptions of other key stake-holders?

Staff within the Aboriginal Health Service engage healthworkers professionally only in staff meetings or other organisational forums—apart from occasional individual discussions about particular clients. Because the healthworkers spend about half their time visiting clients at home, their interactions with doctors, nurses, social workers and other staff members located on-site are restricted. Nevertheless, nearly everyone seems to have an opinion about healthworkers and their practice. It is evident that a significant number of their professional colleagues perceive healthworkers as a potential means to further their own ends.

THE CLIENT'S VIEW

The majority of their clients seem happy to receive home visits from the healthworkers, and generally the relationships appear easy and friendly.

Most clients express a sincere appreciation of the home-visiting service. While many say healthworker services are broadly 'OK', some are enthusiastic: 'wonderful care … I almost feel guilty they look after me so well'; and 'the best thing ever'. Clients express appreciation for Family Care 'helping' them, and some feel particular gratitude for the clinical monitoring: 'If you are an asthmatic, there are people coming out and seeing if you are OK'.

Home visits are particularly valued, as they enable clients to avoid travel into the AHS clinic. One client explained that she is grateful for home visits because she can only move slowly; she has trouble judging the speed of cars, has difficulty crossing the road and is unwilling to use public transport. The health service is accessible to her only through home visits and the provision of transport.

Another client outlines the time-saving advantages of home visits:

> Now, six o'clock this morning, I showered and had me breakfast, and got ready to be picked up and brought in here [to the AHS]. And by the time I get over the treatment, and get back home, what time—it could be another half hour, maybe, so what would that be? It will be about half-past eleven—that's five and a half hours just to get the dressing done … [In contrast], they come to the home—she can do it in forty minutes … To just bring me in here to wash my foot and do a bit of dressing, that's just not on. It used to happen before—y'know I lose time, they lose time, some blokes have to pick me up and bring me back, all those little things y'know.

This client perceives no qualitative difference in the capacity of the health personnel who attend him. Comparing nurses and healthworkers, he suggests:

> They're no better than each other—and some are bloody not the best. You've got to, y'know, tell them what to do—and they don't like being told by the patient.

However, he does emphasise the advantage of having an Aboriginal person look after him:

There is a fair bit of difference, because when they come to my home, they come there and sit down and they fit in easily. They sit down and do their work—bit of a relaxed atmosphere—but you get a white nurse that comes from [the Community Nursing Agency], they don't know whether to ... I've had one old woman there who's [been] there for twenty-nine years, and then she was put out on the truck, from [the Community Nursing Agency] a few years ago. It was like this—I don't know if it was the gaping big hole in my foot, or the colour of my skin was affecting her, but yeah, she had to be eating chocolate, or drinking hot coffee to stimulate her. So, y'know, there's something wrong with [her]. So y'know, you have two different types of people.

Other clients also express appreciation about receiving services specifically from an Aboriginal service provider:

It is good to have healthworkers from the same culture and know they are coming every week.

It is very good for [an Aboriginal]—talking to your own people.

In particular, clients place value on healthworkers accompanying them to appointments with health professionals outside the AHS and on maintaining an overview of the client's health status: '[She] takes me to the surgery—so she knows what's going on between me and the doctors'.

Most express approval for central aspects of healthworker practice, in particular the care and monitoring, the linking or acting as middleman, and the advocacy and emotional support.

THE DOCTOR'S VIEW

Despite obtaining the seal of approval from the clients, doctors within the AHS, who provide general practice services to Family Care clients, express serious concerns about these very activities. Concern about clients' progress motivates their interest in healthworker services. While client consultations with doctors take place predominantly within the medical clinic, those with healthworkers occur mainly at home. The differences in service delivery parallel those in location and in organisation. The doctors have no line-management links with the healthworkers. Physical and organisational distance and associated communication problems magnify misgivings and doubts among doctors about healthworker practice.

Doubts about clinical competence

Few formal procedures link doctors and healthworkers. Only occasionally do healthworkers initiate consultations with doctors, and opportunities for dialogue arise only during meetings or when doctors visit the Family Care office. As doctors rarely accompany healthworkers on home visits, they have limited first-hand experience of healthworker practice.

Most doctors perceive that the central contribution of healthworkers is the collection and provision of information about the community context of the client:

> [The healthworker] has worked brilliantly with me. She explains all the context. She tells me all about the next-door neighbour, what the next-door neighbour is thinking. It's very relevant because the next-door neighbour is the main supporter, and the main complainer, about what's going on, and she knows it all. She knows the background of the family, who's in contact, all that sort of stuff, and it's absolutely vital.

From a colleague's perspective:

> Often one of the very helpful things about the healthworkers is that they know the patient. Especially that's important when a doctor or another member of staff has only just begun to work … Sometimes they can help fill you in on the picture much more quickly than you can get that information from the patient—in terms of more social issues than medical issues.

In brief, doctors report that healthworkers provide important information about the community context of the client. This information encompasses the client's social context—family background, support networks, availability of carers, need for special assistance—and the client's environmental context—type of housing, condition of housing, number of occupants, cooking and storage facilities, washing and sanitation arrangements.

While one doctor values the capacity of healthworkers to provide information about the community context, he expresses doubts about their level of skill, particularly their clinical competence:

> What they are good at is identifying when the patient does have a need … they are good at recognising other things like social needs, [the need for] carers pensions, disability support pensions, those sorts of things, and bringing them in for that. Or when they are quite sick, they're quite good at that … But there again, I'm not sure that those skills are much different from what they had even before they did their healthworker training. It doesn't appear that [they understand clinical indicators]—just a little note saying his blood pressure has been X or his blood pressure has been Y—y'know, no communication about what they are finding.

This doctor suggests that the scope of healthworker practice is limited to the identification of problems and to client transportation. There is no acknowledgement that a healthworker may not only recognise a client's need, but also act independently to resolve it. This absence, and a perceived weakness in healthworkers' clinical skills, leads the doctor to question the quality of their training. This view matches healthworker perceptions that doctors are unaware of their activities in the community context and do not value their qualifications.

Most doctors identify the clinical screening of clients—whether at the clinic or during a home-visit—as a central task of healthworkers:

> The healthworkers in the clinic seem to be mostly involved with screening—doing basic examinations, blood pressure, weights,

heights, things like that, and some of the healthworkers appear to be equipped to give injections. They do seem to be able to do dressings … my experience in the clinic is that it's fairly basic nursing observation … My experience in Family Care is, in fact, that the Family Care healthworkers are doing much the same thing in the home environment.

While screening within the clinic, the clinic healthworker records observations directly into the client's medical file for the immediate information of the doctor. However, the Family Care healthworkers record client information in separate office files to which doctors have no easy access:

We don't actually liaise very greatly. I've been out to do home visits a couple of times with the healthworkers, but I feel there needs to be a lot more liaison between Family Care and the medical clinic … The only information that we have on file that indicates that a patient is a Family Care client is that it is written on the front of the file. We don't have any information that's generated by the Family Care people.

The doctors consider screening to be an important healthworker task, and express concern and frustration that the information generated by Family Care healthworkers rarely reaches them. One doctor emphasises the lack of systematic organisational procedures to ensure the transfer of client information from Family Care to the clinic:

Neither Family Care nor the doctors have seriously sat down and looked at actually setting [a policy] down, and following it through, and making sure that communication has been set up on a systematic, proper basis.

This lack of information not only frustrates doctors, but also fosters doubts about the capacity of healthworkers to interpret clinical observations:

I'm not sure whether they understand why they are doing some of those things—blood pressure and blood sugars—because if they are not reporting on them … I'm not sure how much they can manage them on their own.

In turn, these doubts about the clinical competence of health-workers engender doubts about their capacity to complete other tasks, for instance, client follow-up, maintenance of preventive monitoring schedules and provision of health education. Some doctors suggest that rather than drawing on their own initiative, healthworkers relate only passively to clients. One offers her perception of effective healthworker practice:

A lot of their time is actually wasted monitoring people who are sick and not getting any better, whereas they should be taking an active part in actually improving health. That would be really why they should be visiting—to make sure the sugar is staying good and reinforcing the message for the client about diet and exercise and remembering their tablets, and things like that, rather than just taking their tablets when they run out and taking a blood sugar, which the client often doesn't know why it's being done.

A colleague suggests:

I think we might be able to point the healthworker in the direction of what further needs to be done, because often I'm not sure they're aware of all the different medical problems. My impression is that their focus is on blood pressure and blood sugars, and of course there's lots of other things, like screening, mammography, regular Pap smears, y'know, the preventive work.

The latter comment suggests that doctors should provide health-workers with clinical supervision. However, such an arrangement would entail a major restructure of clinical responsibility. The existing organi-sational structure provides for the clinical supervision of Family Care healthworkers by the Family Care field nurse. It is her responsibility to maintain an overview of client progress and to monitor related healthworker practice.

In short, while doctors appreciate the social and cultural knowledge of healthworkers, they express doubts about their clinical understandings. Because healthworkers rarely consult doctors about patients' abnormal clinical indicators, the doctors perceive that they are unaware of the meaning and implications of abnormal clinical readings. Because of this perceived inaction, some doctors cast doubt on the healthworkers' ability to provide health education and prevention activities.

Concerns about continuity of clinical care

Doctors express concerns about the capacity of healthworkers to follow up the conditions of clients. These concerns arise from the relatively rare occasions when doctors read the Family Care client files. They report little evidence of healthworkers referring clients with sustained high blood pressure or blood sugar levels:

> One high blood pressure reading is not a huge issue, but regular high blood pressure readings is an issue, and … the same with blood sugar readings … Regular high sugar readings are a matter of concern and need to be brought to the attention of the doctor. My feeling's been that fairly frequently that hasn't been the case— in Family Care anyway.

According to another doctor:

> There seems to be a lack of knowledge about when a doctor needs to be called about a blood pressure, and at what stage should a blood sugar be reported. Is it OK to go on taking a 17 [blood sugar level reading] week after week and not doing anything?

In reporting on the extraordinary follow-up efforts by one healthworker, a doctor attributes it to prior hospital experience:

She keeps me informed on a regular basis, verbally. She follows up on things. She is very conscientious and I wonder to what extent it's got to do with her long experience in some sort of other clinical setting … I reckon in a hospital you learn that.

While doctors query the level of follow-up for abnormal clinical readings, they also express concern about the follow-up of the client group in general. One suggests that the particular client group requires an extraordinary commitment to follow up:

The patients in themselves are extremely high follow-up-responsibility type patients. There are very few we can really say, 'See you in a week', and you can have a good gut feeling that they will be back in a week. Whereas in a non-Aboriginal setting, there's a much higher response to, 'See you in a week'. You *will* see them in a week.

Another doctor highlights the unsettled nature of the client group and the need for careful follow-up, observing that clients are subject to constant social pressure and that regular contact with a healthworker supports self-management of illness:

There are clients who are willing and able to monitor their own sugars, or have a partner or a family member who can do it. Unfortunately I know more people with broken glucometers than actually have ones that are working and being utilised—so I think for many people it just seems like another pressure. For people with chronic illness, that regular contact with a health care worker—who can hopefully reinforce the message of the significance of taking their tablets and watching their diet etc.—is probably really good.

The AHS doctors emphasise healthworker follow-up with local general practitioners (GPs). They indicate that most clients also attend consultations with a GP in their own neighbourhood. In particular, they stress the need for healthworkers to follow up with local GPs concerning client medications:

> I think a lot of liaison needs to be done, between the Family Care worker and us, with the local GP—because a lot of these people are in a fairly stable home environment, and they have a local doctor. And that's an issue with the prescription writing ... you need a clear list of the medications ... Sometimes the patient will go to hospital and the discharge letter is only sent to the doctor who sent them to hospital, who may be the local GP ... Their medications could have been changed, or a new diagnosis might have been made ... Certainly most of the people who come here also have a local doctor.

Often local GPs prescribe medications for clients or receive updates of medication changes in client hospital discharge notes without informing the AHS doctors. In order to prevent problems of polypharmacy, the AHS doctors suggest it is necessary for healthworkers to undertake this follow-up.

According to some doctors, poor communication exists between healthworkers and clients about medications. Doctors express concerns because of the potentially dangerous consequences of polypharmacy. One doctor suggests that healthworkers ask conversational questions rather than strategic probing questions central to a client's medical condition:

> Like you can say to a patient, 'You OK with your medications?' and they'll say, 'Yeah, I'm alright'. And *then* you find they haven't been taking them for months, that's why they've got plenty of them at home. Or 'I just don't like them', or 'I don't take them when I'm drinking', 'I don't know what they're for'—all those sorts of other attitudes.

In brief, doctors perceive that healthworkers display a lack of attention to follow-up in three related areas: 1) working closely with clients to address clinical conditions, by encouraging them to adopt relevant preventive health practices and monitoring their medications for the prevention of polypharmacy; 2) follow-up with local GPs in order to monitor medication schedules; 3) follow-up with the AHS doctors concerning clinical problems.

The potential of clinic consultations

Most doctors believe that attendance at their consultations with clients will enable healthworkers to learn more about the client's clinical problems, and that more effective follow-up will result:

> I think it would be very useful for the healthworkers to come with the patients to the consultation … because often they are elderly and sometimes confused, and they're not clear about medications, or what's being given, or whether there is a dossette box for administration of the tablets, and how often the healthworker is visiting, or how often the tablets are being administered … Often they're on lots of different medications because they've got lots of different medical problems.

However, this rarely happens, prompting one doctor to observe:

> Sometimes I see patients who are old, with multiple problems, and who are really demented. They are not able to tell you coherently, 'This is the last person I saw' or what the problems are. The Family Care worker brings them in but leaves them—maybe it's logistics—but leaves them, so I see the patient alone. I get a bit frustrated.

The 'logistics' is the operations of Family Care. The organisation of healthworker caseloads within Family Care has no relation to the operation of the clinic, and there are no formal communication protocols between the clinic and Family Care. Attendance at client medical consultations is not a specified duty for healthworkers, due to their commitments in the field.

Despite 'logistics', the doctors identify significant advantages in the attendance of healthworkers at consultations. They suggest that attendance would enhance the doctor's comprehension of the client's story, provide a more comprehensive background on client medications and enable greater clinical understanding of the client by the healthworker. Significantly, one doctor suggests that it would enable healthworkers to become 'partners' in the provision of clinical care:

> The only way healthworkers can be a partner with doctors here in the clinic, in providing care to that person, is to attend the consult with that patient and understand what went on—what the follow-up is and what the plan is.

Others suggest that lack of confidence and concerns about their 'place' or professional status are factors affecting healthworkers' attendance at consultations:

> I wonder whether it's confidence—it's knowing your role and your place … When there's a problem, the healthworker I'm sure knows there's a problem, and knows this is an important consult—and those are the consults where it's really important for the healthworker to be here with the client.

This reluctance to approach doctors reflects a lack of confidence in their knowledge of health issues, according to another doctor:

> Some health care workers approach us a lot and some don't, and I think it is to do with how much confidence they have in their own decision making. So they might think that we'll think they're silly if they ask, so they don't ask … I think they're affected by the expectation that they should know … The doctors don't expect them to know, and in fact the healthworkers would be amazed how much new doctors here ask the other doctors for help.

Another doctor claims that the (higher) professional status of doctors makes them somewhat unapproachable:

I like to think that I'm approachable … but in fact I might not be, even though I think I am. But that might be one issue—professionally there might be just a whole stereotype about doctors being unapproachable.

Co-ordination through clinical oversight

The co-ordination of client care is of considerable importance to healthworkers, who perceive that their knowledge of the community context is highly relevant. Nevertheless, most doctors consider that it is the doctor's role to co-ordinate client care:

GPs such as myself, we see ourselves as co-coordinators of care. That's the way I understand [it]—in fact it'd be actually written into the official definition of a general practitioner.

Paradoxically, the same doctor suggests that 'practically speaking' healthworkers co-ordinate most Family Care client services:

I recognise that practically speaking, most of the co-ordination of care for a lot of these patients is by the Family Care [health]worker … Probably the ideal is that the GP is co-co-ordinator of care, but delegating much of the responsibility to the health care worker … The GP's role should be very short—in little bursts from time to time … I don't think that we are at that ideal point at the moment. I don't think the healthworkers understand how much we can work together.

The ideal arrangement for the co-ordination of client care, according to this doctor, is that the doctor maintains medical oversight and has final authority, but delegates day-to-day responsibility to the healthworker.

Another approach proposed is that healthworkers 'partner' the doctor in clinical care and the development of a client care plan:

The only way healthworkers can be partners with doctors here in the clinic in providing care to that person is to attend the consult with that patient and understand what went on, what the follow-up is and what the plan is … It may be better if the healthworkers developed their own care plan and it was supplemented by someone else … attending consults and moulding your care plan to whatever's the most recent medical issue.

Both these doctors regard a full understanding by healthworkers of the medical condition of a client as a prerequisite to partnership in the development of care plans and the co-ordination of client care.

Another medical colleague stresses that it is the doctor's responsibility to co-ordinate client care and the healthworker's responsibility to book and regularly attend consultations with the doctor. This doctor perceives that any involvement of healthworkers in client management implies a clinical supervision role by doctors:

[The healthworkers] should know that they're expected [to consult with the doctor]. In other words, we are going to be expecting them to come and talk about their clients … We'd like to know every three months how a client's going … Certainly I would encourage the healthcare workers to make a booking of an hour somewhere or other and bring their client files across and discuss their management … I think the healthcare workers should be liaising more—in which case they could take a more active part in management because they would know more what they're trying to achieve.

In brief, doctors perceive that both they and healthworkers have a significant role in the co-ordination of client care. Whether advocating a partnership or a subordinate role for healthworkers, all doctors perceive that it is their responsibility to maintain clinical oversight. In general, they perceive that co-ordination of care should include the clinical supervision of healthworkers by doctors.

One doctor recognises, however, that high client demand constrains them from supervising healthworkers:

I've often handed things to healthworkers and haven't followed up as much as I've needed to—to know the outcomes really happened.

But it's a pretty tiring experience to do that … In a way, patients have got so many problems or whatever—to actually start supervising the healthworker as much as the patient, it just adds immeasurably to the responsibility.

A doctor with an involvement in an outreach healthworker programme at another site proposes an alternative model. At the other site, coherent strategies and clear expectations support healthworkers and enable them to take responsibility and to follow up on issues. This works for both the healthworkers and the doctors:

There's been a clear coherent strategy, there's been a long-term plan, and there have been regular meetings—and that's been really satisfactory. The [health]workers have been placed in a position of responsibility, have clear expectations, and really pick up on all sorts of issues and follow through and are clearly very competent. That's in a programme where structurally they're set up to succeed—in contrast to other programmes which weren't well written from the beginning and go through frequent changes. So that's what makes me think it's structural issues and unclear expectations and uncertainty about roles [that inhibit healthworker effectiveness].

This doctor indicates that both supervision and feedback are structured into the programme:

It's expected that they will have that supervision every week, where they talk about patients and issues that are arising. And it's also expected they will feed back to the doctors. So you've essentially got it structured into their work.

In short, this doctor recognises that effective programmes with healthworkers in positions of responsibility require clear role definitions, clear expectations, goal-centred tasks and clearly defined structures for supervision. Consequently, she perceives that a planned and structured protocol of supervision is fundamental.

Scepticism about clinical training

Linked to doctors' proposals to supervise healthworkers is scepticism about their clinical competence. In large measure, doctors attribute these deficits to inadequate training.

While doctors perceive that some healthworkers are competent in clinical observation, the description of presenting problems, monitoring medications and dressing wounds, most express doubts about the rigour of healthworker training:

> I feel as though we have not given Aboriginal healthworkers sufficient education or training—not just training theoretically but practical supervision, really enabling type of education where they don't just know it, they do it, and they're regularly checked that they can do it and they can understand it … There's a one-off—they get this big dose and that's supposed to get them through whatever happens next, get them into any job, and I don't think it works that way.

Another doctor suggests that healthworkers need more training in the area of medications and a deeper understanding of the medical risks of polypharmacy and non-adherence:

> There are skills they could and should have, but I think in practice it doesn't work out that way … Awareness of the importance of the issue, for example, polypharmacy and the risks to the patient, or the risks of non-compliance—the awareness of the importance of the issue … I think it really comes down to critical thinking, a critical approach and a strong sense of where they can intervene to improve health.

This doctor proposes that as well as clinical understandings and ability to intervene, healthworkers require sophisticated investigative skills:

> [Healthworkers need the] ability or skill to raise [concerns] on a regular basis with the patient—the skill in questioning, the skill in

non-directive questioning and also direct questioning, which allow patients to speak the truth, [the] ability to not take answers completely at face value, and to learn to ask questions in roundabout ways … Now I say things like, 'What medications are you on?' and they can't name them. 'Do you know what they're for?', and often they don't know what they're for. 'Do you sometimes forget to take the morning one, or the night one?' 'Oh yeah'. 'Do you sometimes forget to take the midday one?'—a lot of people forget that one, and they'll say, 'I never take it'. That sort of thing.

Another doctor regards healthworker training as too general and proposes further specialised training:

They don't have very much specialised knowledge of any of the things they need to do for health promotion. So for instance, I worked with the women's health care worker, who was a qualified health care worker, but basically we just really had to start from scratch, and presumably it happens in other areas as well— sexually transmitted diseases, needle exchange … They have no specific knowledge in any of the fields that they're working in … I think people probably need a bit of in-service.

Some doctors cite the advantages of experience and training within a structured and supervised hospital setting:

In a hospital you learn that if you don't do things, you get in trouble. That might be part of it—if you don't follow up on something that's important, there is a consequence … It's a sort of a structured setting and a supervised setting … I think it helps to give them a competent sense of responsibility, in some sort of way.

Another advantage of a hospital setting, according to one doctor, is that it provides an awareness of the division of labour in health and the opportunity to understand the training of nurses and other health professionals. Comparing healthworkers and nurses, a doctor observes:

> I don't get as much feedback from the community nurses as I would like either. I very rarely get much feedback there, but I have a sense that there's more awareness in nursing to attention and follow-through [compared with healthworkers].

This doctor suggests that doctors and nurses become familiar with their respective professions during their training in hospitals and develop mutual trust in the process. In contrast, healthworkers remain an unknown quantity, as doctors lack familiarity with their training:

> [I'm] not particularly [familiar with the training]. I know that they go to [Aboriginal Healthworker College], and I know they do some practical work as well …

> [I'm] not very aware. I hear some of the talk, and pick up on some of the jargon, but not very aware of what it actually involves—even what competencies or what. 'Cause I hear some discussion about immunisation or essential medications and that—and healthworkers can't do this, this and this 'cause they're not covered and all that, but I've never sorted out the details of that.

One doctor perceives that industry expectations concerning the capacity of healthworkers is far too high:

> At this point, I think that, basically I think there's an expectation on healthworkers that they can actually do a lot more than they're actually trained to do, and that they actually know a lot more than they're actually seen to know—about everything. And I think there should be recognition with healthworkers, as there is with doctors, that in fact when you graduate you've basically licensed to learn, and the first year out should be on-the-job training. People shouldn't expect them to do things unless they've been shown, and there should be a fair degree of supervision and instruction.

In brief, the doctors perceive deficits in two broad areas of health-worker training. The content of the training lacks coverage of critical understandings related to the effects of medications, investigative communication skills and knowledge of specialised areas of health. The organisation of the training lacks ongoing professional development opportunities and practical hands-on training experiences. The doctors suggest that the structured and supervised setting of a hospital has advantages as a training setting, particularly for the development of clinical skills and the capacity to follow up, and for strengthening professional relationships.

THE SUPPORT STAFF VIEW

The Welfare and Transport sections of the AHS both have links with Family Care healthworkers and their clients. The situation of staff in both sections is similar to that of AHS doctors: most are distant from the day-to-day activities of Family Care. Generally, welfare and transport workers view healthworkers in terms of their potential to provide specific services. In other words, common to both is a perception that healthworkers could provide greater assistance to their own programmes.

The Welfare section offers a range of social services to Aboriginal clients, including direct emergency relief by way of financial assistance, food parcels and blankets; advocacy for negotiating payment of outstanding rent, electricity, gas, water and phone accounts; assistance with the organisation of funerals; provision of accommodation and housing advocacy. Unlike Family Care, it provides services primarily from within the AHS office. In order to receive assistance, clients must attend an appointment.

Four permanent workers, with help from volunteers, provide the welfare services. While one of the permanent staff regularly assists a Family Care healthworker with male clients, others have negligible experience alongside healthworkers. Predominantly, client housing needs and cases requiring emergency welfare assistance bring Family Care healthworkers into contact with Welfare staff. Despite their limited experience of working with healthworkers, the welfare workers have numerous suggestions concerning healthworker activities.

According to one welfare worker, while healthworker services in the community are beneficial in themselves, of equal value is the reduction in client demand at the AHS—home visits result in less pressure on clinic doctors to treat minor ailments. This worker also believes that healthworkers should supplement applications for government welfare assistance with the necessary medical documentation.

In contrast to the accounts of doctors, another welfare worker indicates that the healthworkers' main contribution is facilitating the contact between the frail-aged and disabled clients and 'white' doctors:

> You won't see many [Aboriginal] doctors. It's good people have healthworkers as a first point of contact, it eases their contact with white doctors. Clients will really speak to an Aboriginal healthworker or an Aboriginal nurse.

While welfare workers are largely ignorant of the relationship between healthworkers and doctors, most acknowledge the link between healthworkers and the community.

A link to the community

One welfare worker suggests that the healthworkers' general overview of the health of the Aboriginal community is of great value. In her view, because healthworkers refer clients to Welfare, they also provide the Welfare section with a presence in the community. She emphasises the pivotal nature of their outreach role:

> They've got such good liaison with the community. See not everyone comes in for help. The way the welfare agency is structured here, you've got to actually come in and make an appointment … They're out there seeing things, yeah, I think that's the benefit of their role, y'know—apart from all the other issues, like being so close to the community and having a good network and everything. The fact that they go out to people I think is hugely [important] … they see a lot more of what's going on.

This worker suggests that Aboriginal healthworkers have a unique overview of their community's needs. She perceives that their understanding of problems extends far beyond the information conveyed by clients who attend the AHS. She observes that healthworkers offer vital support to combat widespread despair:

> A lot of people give up, I think. The level of depression and hopelessness is quite extreme. That's why I think healthworkers have got a very big role ... I think they do recognise the degree of hopelessness, they are very good in that. I think they are a huge support.

However, she also proposes that healthworkers fail to effectively address housing problems. She believes that inadequate housing is the cause of many health problems:

> There's a lot of deaths and illnesses associated with the housing, I reckon. I'm just seeing it here. I mean, I'm not making that as the scientific statement, but you can see it, day by day, how bad it is ... A lot of the babies who've died this year—I think practically every mother's been homeless that I can think of, apart from one, and there the child was grossly overcrowded, like grossly overcrowded, and partly the death seemed to be related to that ...
>
> I think the housing problem amongst Aboriginal communities overwhelms everyone a bit—it's so extreme ... Every house that the healthworker would go to, there would be a housing problem—other people staying, or staying off and on, or the younger family member who can't get housing, or even an older family member, or can't get appropriate housing ...

If healthworkers were given more training, this welfare worker suggests, it would increase their capacity to recognise and act when overcrowding is actually a situation of homelessness:

> I think the [healthworkers] are very good, but I do think probably they could have more sort of input about housing issues … Quite often families are actually homeless, and probably, y'know, I think the healthworker training needs to make sure that people are very alert to that, and sort of detect it. Like they go to so many of these overcrowded houses, y'know, it could be part of their role to see that the families are actually homeless, not 'overcrowding', and direct them to housing agencies … They need to know who those agencies are … know how to advocate to them, and that the clients will be eligible—and try and put pressure on to see if they can get them housed.

She observes that because the healthworkers are familiar with the community context, they are more informed on housing issues than most health professionals:

> People are more willing to tell a healthworker they're homeless than a specialist at [the Children's Hospital]. And that's where I really do think there's a huge breakdown—y'know. The specialists talk to the patients as though they're housed, and most of the time, as you well know, they're not.

Nevertheless, one of her colleagues points out that the existing load on healthworkers is already substantial.

'It takes a lot of your altruism'

A male welfare worker who assists a healthworker with the care of male clients perceives that healthworkers face a large, difficult and complex task. He recognises the extensive social issues that confront healthworkers in the community, the need for a holistic approach and, notably, the consequences when clear guidelines are lacking:

> I think that's what's really much harder—because they provide a bigger service … I think that's what wears people out, because its really hard to provide a service in the community with a limited

staff ... Y'know, I think when you're out there in the community right, and you're dealing with like the aged, right, who really tend to stress you out sometimes—because you're looking at people that's really aged and chronic, and it takes out a lot of your altruism ... I think that's what burns people out, and sometimes I see it myself ... they do get burnt up.

This worker observes that healthworkers put in sustained effort due to the mobility and dependency of clients:

Y'know, if you're trying to provide a service for the community, and if you're to see a client in the morning and the client's not there, right, and then you have to re-schedule everything you have, then to work around it. You have to go back to see the client again ... some people I guess are so dependent on the healthworker to do so much for them—they kind of like burn them out because there's a big need out there in the community.

In his perception, healthworkers provide a 'bigger' service: one that requires a large investment of energy due to the range of client needs, their dependence and their other priorities. For instance, he cites the effort required in filling a prescription for a client:

Even with the [medication] scripts sometimes, I mean it's not like you just pick up a script ... you actually have to bring the script in, make sure you get it across the street, make sure it's filled out, and make sure you get it back the next day, plus get it to the chemist and pick it up. There's a lot of work involved ... and that's where, I think that's where the burning out comes out with the healthworker sometimes.

His understanding of the context of healthworker practice enables this welfare worker to acknowledge the complexities within the apparently simple task of filling a prescription. He notes that the task is set in a context of dependency and that the act of service provision in itself is very likely to create further demands. He also recognises that stress is an inevitable outcome for healthworkers and that their potential for 'burnout' requires management.

This worker recognises that healthworker practice requires a significant emotional investment. Amidst constant stress and the threat of burnout, he observes that healthworkers relieve stress by chatting and joking together in the office:

> I think every one has their own way of relieving stress ... Y'know, I go out there sometimes and people say, 'Oh, y'know, we go over to Family Care and all those girls are just sitting around', y'know. I mean like I'm, 'Well what do you want them to do? What do you expect them to do?' I mean they're in the office relaxing, right, and you can't say how much time they actually spent out on the road. They don't know they're actually taking a break from all the stress of driving back and forth.

Workers in the Transport section perceive healthworker strategies for relieving stress quite differently. Located in the main AHS building, the Transport section comprises four drivers and a manager. All staff are male, four Aboriginal and one non-Aboriginal. The manager is responsible for the maintenance of the whole AHS fleet of vehicles and co-ordinates the transport of clients to and from the AHS. As all AHS cars are on call to the Transport manager, a healthworker in the field can be called on her mobile phone and requested to transport a client.

The Family Care budget funds one of the staff positions in the Transport section, specifically to ensure the ready availability of transport for their clients. Previously, the Family Care driver operated from within the Family Care section, and consequently he knows more about healthworker activities than his colleagues. This is his view of the healthworker role:

> They're just somebody who goes out to people's houses, and they just keep an eye on their sickness or whatever ... They do most of

their work out in the field in the first line ... make sure their tablets are right, make sure they're taking the right dosage and not overdosing themselves ... They just do all their work in the home, y'know ... they go out and do dressings, blood pressure, sugar levels, things like that—just check on whether they're going OK, socially and healthy-wise like.

Both the Transport manager and the Family Care driver recognise that professional boundaries limit the practice of healthworkers: 'Like they can't do injections unless a registered nurse is there ... They only can go so far.' Upon reflection, the Transport manager observes that, in general, Transport staff are uninformed about the healthworker role:

I think we only focus on what we see here actually. We probably don't really know ... what they should be doing, how far they should be going. We're only thinking of what we think they should be—how far they're meant to go. We've never been told what they've been [employed to do].

Nevertheless, when ferrying clients, Transport drivers often receive complaints about healthworkers.

Complaining clients

According to the Family Care driver, clients often complain that healthworkers complete only part of their task, miss scheduled visits or fail to deliver medications in a timely manner:

Like I do a lot of driving and like I pick up the complaints of all these people sometimes. 'They never come out to see me this week', 'They didn't come out for two weeks', 'I haven't seen them for three weeks'—and every time they ring in for something, they say it takes a day and a half before they even get what they want, like a script or something.

The driver also reports that some clients complain about the content and value of home visits, and he thinks the healthworkers should spend more time with clients:

> Some of them say, 'Oh yeah, they come out here and test my sugar and that, but what for though? They don't tell nothin' about it. They don't say, "You're doing well" or … they could say, "Don't eat that food so much now" … They just say, "Aw, it's goin' OK", and that's it … [The clients] are not that educated, half of 'em that they go and see, but they should explain it to 'em … I just reckon they need to have more contact with their clients … if they see they're feeling a bit down or whatever, hang around a while.

The Transport manager claims that the failure of healthworkers to visit clients creates extra work for Transport staff, and the drivers perceive substantial deficiencies in the operations of healthworkers:

> We get a lot of complaints from their clients that they don't see them, so they ring us up about two o'clock saying, 'Can you pick us up so we can go and see a doctor' or 'get our tablet box filled'.

Healthworkers 'fall short'

The drivers also express concerns about healthworkers from their own observations. For example, some worry about the frailty of many clients and suggest that healthworkers should accompany frail clients to and from their outside (non AHS) medical consultations:

> With the high priority patients, say somebody who needs someone to be with them, I don't think they should drop them off and leave them at a hospital. I reckon they should sit with them at the hospital—like say, if it's a client like Annie, y'know, wheelchair bound, stay around with them and make sure they're right and that they get home OK, instead of like ringing up and saying, 'OK, he's ready at [the General Hospital] now, I've got to go over here. Can someone come over and pick her up?' Whereas I reckon they should drop them off and then go to wherever they have to go to.

The Transport manager also thinks that healthworkers should wait with their clients at the clinic—a view similar to those expressed by doctors. He sees the provision of home care by healthworkers as having the potential to ease the burden on both the Transport section and (echoing a welfare worker above) the clinic:

> 'Cause that could save a lot of time on bringing some clients in here—they could go out there. You get clients coming in here, well we had some come in for two weeks, every day, just for a flu. And I thought, well … healthworkers [have] been trained, they should be able to do that out there, do a dressing out there instead of bringing them in here every day. Saves a lot of time.

All these comments from staff whose primary job is to transport clients contrast sharply, even ironically, with those of other stakeholders with their own special interests. The welfare workers think the health-workers could do more to assist welfare and housing issues, the doctors think they could do more to assist clinical management, and the trans-port workers think they could reduce the burden of demand by treating more patients at home. They all perceive a large degree of flexibility or plasticity in the healthworker role.

Transport workers also propose that it would assist them if health-workers were more available on their mobile phones, even on home visits:

> They're hard to contact. It's hard to give a really good service when they got their mobile phones in the car [during a home visit]. You can't get hold of them when you need to. A couple of times they needed to be contacted to go out and see a client while they're out in the suburbs, and then they'll turn around, and 'cause you can't contact them—they won't answer that phone till an hour later—and in this time they've probably gone … and it's too late to go back there.

They also express concerns about transporting medications to clients, a job they identify as the responsibility of a healthworker. The Family

Care driver suggests that if healthworkers maintain the full complement of client medications through regular home visits, then requests for Transport drivers to deliver medications will cease. He considers that, in general, the healthworkers are not working to full capacity:

> You see, they say they got, say, six or seven clients a day, right, and they're coming back here at twelve o'clock and they're leaving here at ten o'clock. I want to know what they've done in that time. It doesn't seem like they would have done too much to provide a service or improve the lifestyle of these people in the home who are wheelchair bound, or just single and haven't got any other family support, anything like that round them … And I don't see anything productively done in that service over there in the afternoons. There's a lot of sitting around and just talking—communicatin' … I notice they do a lot of talking over there, and I don't see much work being done.

While the welfare worker suggests that sitting and chatting is a crucial opportunity for healthworkers to debrief and relax, the Family Care driver interprets this as evidence that they are not working to full capacity. In his estimation, they 'fall short':

> I reckon it's good that they go round to people's houses and they do their thing [but] they don't completely fulfil their services that they are meant to provide. They fall short on them now and again … one week they'll go to a client and then next week they won't even see them, they won't even go there at all.

In conclusion, while Transport staff have a reasonably clear understanding of the narrow clinical services offered by Family Care healthworkers, they report that they have never really been informed about the healthworker role. When they transport Family Care clients to the clinic, the drivers frequently receive complaints about the shortcomings of the healthworkers, and find that the clients' views support their own observations of healthworkers as 'just sitting around talking in the office'. According to the drivers, the healthworkers fall short of their potential, and should make greater efforts to accompany clients to medical consultations both within the AHS and with other providers.

According to most staff in the Welfare section, healthworkers play an important role as the outreach workers for the AHS. They suggest that healthworkers stimulate awareness within the AHS of community needs, provide essential and accessible emotional support to the community and, to a degree, give the Welfare section a community presence.

Both Transport and Welfare staff perceive various ways that the healthworkers could be of more assistance to their own programmes. The Transport workers suggest that if the healthworkers were more easily contactable in the field, they could transport more clients, and that if they provided more comprehensive services to clients at home, clients would not require transport to the AHS. The Welfare workers suggest that healthworkers should assist them more by extending client access to Welfare housing services.

However, one Welfare worker with experience of working alongside a healthworker recognises the complexities they face in the community, sees that they are vulnerable to 'burnout', and defends the strategies they use to relieve stress on their return to the office.

THE NURSE'S VIEW

The AHS employs nurses in a variety of roles and settings. Within Family Care, a registered nurse fills the field nurse position. She provides day-to-day clinical support and supervision to Family Care healthworkers. Within other sections of the AHS, registered nurses include the clinic co-ordinator within the Medical team, the clinic sister, three community nurses, the team leader of the Health Promotion section, and the deputy director of the AHS. Except for the clinic-co-ordinator and one of the community nurses, all the nurses outside Family Care are Aboriginal.

The intermittent occasions when the activities of healthworkers and nurses coincide provide the basis for the perceptions of 'other AHS nurses'—those in sections of the health service other than Family Care. Primarily, the other AHS nurses undertake activities in the clinic, management duties, health promotion and community outreach to clients who are mainly other than the frail-aged and disabled.

Two broad current issues dominate the perceptions of healthworkers by the 'other AHS nurses'. The first is negotiations between the healthworkers' union and the AHS for a new healthworker award; the second is a promotion of the pivotal role of Aboriginal healthworkers by the state Director of Aboriginal Health and a senior manager within the AHS, linked with preparations for two new outreach programmes. As a result of the heavy emphasis on healthworkers, Aboriginal nurses feel a singular lack of recognition. They view many of the claims about Aboriginal healthworkers as not only excessive, but also dismissive of their own contribution to Aboriginal health.

Why the 'big emphasis' on healthworkers?

Most of the 'other AHS nurses' admit they have little hands-on experience of working with Family Care healthworkers. Neither are they particularly clear about either the extent or specifics of healthworker activities. An Aboriginal nurse summarises their perceptions:

> There is confusion, according to people in the organisation, about the role of the healthworker and the role of the registered nurse, and I think that's very obvious to people who've been here—that it's causing a lot of distress, particularly as we have several Aboriginal registered nurses ... I think sometimes people expect too much from healthworkers—they're expected to do nothing and everything!
>
> ... Unless you get a [registration] board that says, 'This is the role of the healthworker', it's very difficult. 'Cause people expect them to do and be anything, from being basically just a taxi driver in some areas, to doing very specialised clinical skills that even in teaching hospitals would be regarded as very specialist skills. So there's no one role ... people are constantly fighting over the role of the Aboriginal health care worker.

According to this nurse, confusion and conflict exist within the organisation about the role of healthworkers. Her assessment that healthworkers 'are expected to do nothing and everything' echoes Rita's experience of being a Jack of all trades' (see Chapter 2). She identifies an urgent need for a registration board to clearly define the role of healthworkers. In her view, the uncertainty, and a sense that healthworkers have almost equal or perhaps greater status than nurses, causes her and other Aboriginal nurses considerable distress.

Equally disturbing for nurses is the promotion of healthworkers by senior management and the state Director of Aboriginal Health, accompanied by what they perceive as dubious claims about healthworker capacity. Nurses perceive that bureaucratic and management rhetoric within Aboriginal Health places undue emphasis on healthworkers, inflates their importance and exaggerates their competence. The nurses find the assertion that healthworkers could one day replace them outrageous:

> One of the indications is we will be made redundant and the healthworkers take over, y'know. There seems to be this big emphasis on healthworkers, but we're black nurses and we went and did all our training, and y'know, [it] makes it seem as if we mean nothing! ... The healthworkers are the be-all and end-all here in this place, and I've done all this and don't get any recognition! And it is disheartening sometimes. You think, well why am I taking on all this responsibility and going home with a headache?

The claim that healthworkers can replace nurses provokes ridicule from the non-Aboriginal clinic co-ordinator:

> I think there are people in high places ... who see that clinical role [of the healthworker] as totally exaggerated ... [A senior bureaucrat] said that in three years' time there wouldn't be any more registered nurses—healthworkers would have taken over. Now that to me just demonstrates to me that [the speaker] doesn't

actually know a) about what a healthworker wants to do and does; and b) about a corps of registered nurse staff—and the fact that, I mean nursing is an international body!

Another Aboriginal nurse reveals her 'disgust' at what, in her perception, is an attempt to marginalise nurses:

> I always felt there was this thing to remove registered nurses from Aboriginal health … I think it's disgusting, in a nutshell, because Aboriginal healthworkers were never there to take over a profession. It was always to complement it, and to be another professional group—like you have registered nurses, you have Aboriginal health-workers, you have doctors, kind of thing. You don't sort of take out a whole professional group out of the equation, because there are things that nurses do very well, because that's what we've been trained for, from day one … There's a lack of acknowledgment that the registered nurse plays a very important role in primary health care … I mean you recognise that the approaches to the training can be questioned, but you can't question someone's Aboriginality.

In challenging the idea that healthworkers can replace nurses, this nurse also contests an underlying assumption of the proposal: that nursing training alienates Aboriginal people from their own culture. While she thinks it is legitimate to question the training programme of nurses, it is unacceptable to question an Indigenous nurse's Aboriginality. She suggests that nursing and healthworker roles are complementary.

Another Aboriginal nurse queries the distinction between the roles of nurse and healthworker. She proposes that healthworker training was originally a bridge into nursing, but concedes that this thinking has shifted:

> Well, I think the concept of what the healthworker's [training] course is about now, I think it's just gone off track. Originally it was—from my recollection and my own interpretation—I think it was like a bridging course for people to get in to do their enrolled

nursing, and their registered nurse training. That was the original thing I thought was happening.

This example of how the rhetoric concerning healthworkers influences other health professionals is provided by an Aboriginal nurse, who perceives that many embrace the participation of a healthworker and ignore the possibility of collaboration with an Aboriginal nurse or doctor:

> We had the doctor from [the General Hospital] come in here, and he was going to set up this cardiac programme. They were looking at diagnosing and treating people here with stress tests, it was almost like a research. But they were providing everything here, with a specialist, and they were saying how they'd get a healthworker. And I asked whether they understand what a healthworker is. You see, I'm a *health* worker, doctors are *health* workers— so whether they mean a nurse in that context, or whether they actually mean a healthworker. And if they mean an Aboriginal healthworker, you couldn't put a person in that position, because it's a specialised field.

In essence, the 'other AHS nurses', particularly the Aboriginal nurses, indicate that claims about healthworkers are exaggerated, particularly their competence and their importance in the delivery of Aboriginal health services. In comparison, Aboriginal nurses feel a lack of recognition for their own contribution, which extends to their relative remuneration.

One reason for the deployment of primary health workers in the international context is their supposed cost-effectiveness. Ironically, Aboriginal nurses perceive that under a new industrial award, healthworkers will receive too much:

> Looking at the Aboriginal Healthworker's Award, it would be cheaper to employ a registered nurse than it is a healthworker. If they got what they are asking for under this new award—they are

asking for $46,000 per year [level 4.1]—I don't even get that much for three certificates ... I mean, they'll price themselves out of a job.

Another Aboriginal nurse observes:

I mean, look at the salaries for clinical nurses, y'know, nurses with years of experience, and I think the highest you can get to, like actually working in a hospital and being a clinical nurse specialist—around $45,000 ... and healthworkers can get that in a specialist role, too!

Not only do Aboriginal nurses have concerns about healthworker remuneration, but they are angry about a 'specialist' healthworker category in the industrial award. Two suggest that this concept subverts the lexicon of medicine:

When you're doing coronary care, or heart—looking after coronary care patients, intensive care patients, paediatric patients—it's all an extra course. We do three years' training, and then you do another six months specialised training and then you get another certificate—so it's a specialist course ... When I hear that the [healthworker] award [covers specialisations] ... how can you be a specialist in, say heart health, when you've not even done a coronary care course? I mean, I'm not a specialist, and I've got three certificates ... I mean, you're employed as a heart healthworker, but you're not a 'specialist' in that area ... Terminology ... people don't understand what these words mean ... they've got a whole meaning in the medical area.

Her Aboriginal colleague asks:

What do you call specialists? I mean, like a clinical nurse specialist would have to have had ten years' experience in that field of her work to become a midwife—clinical nurse specialist in midwifery.

You'd have to have at least ten years' experience in that field, and what do they have to have?

The Aboriginal nurses perceive that the designation 'specialist' within nursing or medicine is bestowed only on a practitioner with years of clinical training and experience. In comparison to the sophisticated skills of a registered nurse or a clinical nurse specialist, they consider that most healthworkers possess only very basic clinical skills. They are affronted not only by rash statements from the bureaucracy and senior managers that exaggerate the competence and status of healthworkers, but by the distinct possibility of their legitimation within an industrial award.

According to one nurse, the commitment of some managers to healthworkers makes it appear that they are content for clients to receive second-rate care:

> I don't understand why management actually pushes so much for healthworkers to be [the main health service] people … [It's] saying that Aboriginal people aren't clever enough to be in mainstream [nursing] courses … Anywhere else, the healthworker is nothing much but just an assistant of the assistant. You have a registered nurse, and then you have an enrolled nurse, and then there's the healthworker … It's like underselling their people, like saying, 'You're a second-class citizen, you can be looked after by people who've got second-class qualifications'.

This nurse suggests that rather than training Aboriginal people as healthworkers, it would be more effective to train them as enrolled nurses. She observes that the clinical healthworker role is very similar to that of an enrolled nurse, but that enrolled nursing offers more of a career:

> Y'know, most of those [healthworkers] there could do their registered nurse training. If not their registered nurse, they could very easily do their enrolled nurse training—so why not? Why

> have we created this little split? ... If the healthworker is doing clinical work, they're turning them into nursing assistants aren't they, or enrolled nurses. So if this is going to be their role, why don't they just do that, and do a mainstream course. Because think of the bloody benefits, y'know, doing mainstream courses. For one thing, you can pick up your bag and go anywhere and get a job— so in fact it's helpful for people to do it.

She also suggests that the professional discord between nurses and health-workers creates distress for nurses and problems for healthworkers:

> Why have we created this little split? Because of that, the health-workers do not get the support they want and need from registered nurses ... Most registered nurses aren't going to tell them either ... they're all so into protecting their territory.

A perception exists that some nurses are unwilling to support healthworkers in the workplace. As is reported in Chapter 4, this perception is shared by healthworkers.

Competence at the frontline?

While nurses question the competence of healthworkers as the first point of contact with clients, healthworkers perceive that they should occupy this frontline role. However, an Aboriginal nurse observes that in the city, most Aboriginal people prefer to see a doctor:

> You hear this comment that Aboriginal healthworkers are the first person of contact for a lot of people. It might be in the outback, but it's not necessarily so in the city. Talking to people here, if they were sick they'd want to see a doctor. I often get consulted— y'know, 'Look this is happening'—and I'll give them an idea and then they go to see the doctor. But they won't want to see a health-worker ... If you're sick, what can they do?

This nurse suggests that healthworkers lack sufficient clinical credibility with clients either to provide the first point of contact or even to ensure client attendance at the Health Service: 'If you're going to be in that role, where you're going to be bringing people in to see the doctors, you have to be more assertive, you have to be able to convince'.

Another Aboriginal nurse proposes that being the first point of contact in the community requires flexibility rather than clinical competence:

> I don't think you'd be able to address someone's diabetes problem if their most pressing problem was that their son was going to court and could face fifteen years in prison ... I've been involved in that too, where the client's needs are in conflict with what I think their needs should be—but you just have to go with that. I think that's just Aboriginal health really.

Notable is the background context of these two disparate views. The former comment comes from an Aboriginal nurse with considerable experience in the clinical domain; the latter from an Aboriginal nurse with wide experience in the community domain.

However, an Aboriginal community nurse insists that clinical competence and confidence constitute the bottom line in the community context:

> I know community nursing is a lot different ... I think you have to have more, a certain level of clinical skills. If you see a pale flaccid baby at a house, and its temperature's through the roof, and knowing that if this kid isn't taken to some medical—to get help straight away, y'know, make sure that child is taken straight to the doctor, or a hospital preferably ... Seeing that that baby isn't going to make it, y'know, at night time y'know that it'll be going into convulsions and fever, y'know what I mean, and knowing to give it a tepid sponge, not cold, y'know, knowing what to do ... Like if [healthworkers] give immunisations and the baby goes frail, to give adrenalin and put an airway in and resuscitate it, y'know, yeah—that's the bottom line I reckon.

Another nurse highlights the needs of healthworkers for clinical competence and confidence:

> At the one level, there's these ambit claims of the certification, and yet the lack of real, solid training that gives inner confidence … It's like that very wavering self-esteem that's linked to a rather tenuous training … There's a huge difference between healthworkers who have got enrolled nurse training behind them and those who have not … not only in their clinical domain, but in their whole approach to their work—planning … self-regulation, self-sufficiency, adhering to ethical practice, code of ethical practice—because their training is such that it does provide that background. It gives confidence, I think that's the vital factor. It's really not so much the knowledge, it's the confidence and their basic experience. You can't replace actual experience.

Amidst promotional claims from management and bureaucracy, nurses question the concept of healthworkers as first point of client contact. In essence, they suggest that healthworkers lack the necessary clinical competence and confidence for this pivotal role. Most nurses observe a profound difference between the nature of their own training and that of healthworkers.

Training: clinical or preventive?

While they have little detailed knowledge of the healthworker training programme, nurses draw their conclusions from their experiences in the workplace. They suggest that the clinical training is extremely limited. According to one nurse, not only is the training incomplete in fundamental respects but, in the light of exaggerated statements about the capacities of healthworkers, it is abusive:

> People aren't bothering to teach them that sort of systemic approach. On the one hand they're saying these people can do anything, and on the other hand they're giving them a very basic third-class training … Once I went through [the seriousness of a

diabetic's condition] with [two healthworkers]. They said, 'Oh, oh my God!'—they were really worried that they hadn't known [the correct treatment] and had unwittingly put this person in danger … People are saying, 'They can do this, that and the other' … On the other hand, they are not giving them the tools to deal with it, and it is abusive—I think it is a very abusive system.

Like some doctors, nurses advocate for healthworkers to train in a hospital environment, where they can integrate theory and practice, and receive the necessary supervision:

Firstly, [in nursing training] you're taught about things, but also you still do some on-the-job training, y'know … If we'd have something in lectures, somebody telling us about a certain syndrome or illness or something, that was fine, but once I actually got to a person who was sick and had all these things, then I was able to make the connection for myself. This sort of putting together the theory and the practical, and I guess that's what being with sick people does … As your experience grows, and you get that structured supervision and feedback, so does your confidence grow … You start to be able to relate things from observations to one another … and the patterns, which show that they're not satisfactory.

One Aboriginal nurse questions the usefulness of this approach for healthworkers. She perceives that hospital training develops a task focus on curative care, whereas in the community a healthworker needs more client focus, on preventive care:

Nurses are trained to provide clinical nursing, they're trained to look after sick people … You don't get taught how to look after well people, or to keep well people healthy—you become a highly professional person who can work very well in a hospital setting … I think that [point] is important. If you want to work in the community, you can't just walk in and do a dressing for somebody and walk out again, and the whole world is falling down around that person—which is what you are trained in hospitals. And when you go into communities, you have to rethink the way you do things, like you can't just do a task. You become very task-orientated in hospitals—this one has got to have this, and the other one has got to have that—and you look at them as a task you have to do to that person. And so you have to rethink.

Another nurse also questions the focus on the clinical competence of healthworkers, and indicates the need to distinguish between clinical training and training primary health care practitioners:

In the city, you've got people [healthworkers] who are being mod-elled for some reason or another onto being little nurses instead of primary health care practitioners, and I feel that that's a major failing. You either need to get a good solid medical and nursing background with the proper clinical skills, if you are going to prac-tise and call yourself that, and/or get a primary health care set of skills. And at the moment, I feel that [the healthworkers] have got rather an unfortunate incomplete bundle of things that don't really integrate.

This nurse highlights the confusion about the healthworker role. Is it focused primarily on clinical skills and curative care, or is it more holistic and focused primarily on prevention?

In conclusion, while senior managers and bureaucrats promote a piv-otal role for Aboriginal healthworkers, most nurses remain unimpressed. They identify considerable confusion within the organisation about healthworkers who are 'able to do nothing and everything'. Nurses observe that claims made concerning healthworkers are often both uninformed and dubious, and the Aboriginal nurses, in particular, indi-cate that such claims make them feel both unacknowledged and undervalued.

THE FIELD NURSE'S VIEW

In marked contrast to other stakeholders, the Family Care field nurse works closely with healthworkers on a day-to-day basis. The field nurse co-ordinates two major components of the Family Care programme: 1) the initial client assessment and care plan development, and 2) the ongoing monitoring of client progress. The field nurse reviews client files, provides healthworkers with clinical supervision and occasionally accompanies them on home visits.

The field nurse's familiarity with healthworkers and clients gives her a unique insight. Like the many other AHS nurses and doctors, the registered nurses who have filled the field nurse position express concerns about healthworker practice—for instance, their level of clinical skills and capacity to follow up. This section records the perspectives of two field nurses: Karen, a non-Aboriginal nurse who subsequently left on maternity leave, and her predecessor, Jeanne, an Aboriginal nurse. Both acknowledge that the somewhat chaotic context of Aboriginal family life has an enormous impact on healthworker practice.

The field nurse has a supervisory relationship with healthworkers, and Karen describes her view of this role:

> Where there are things I'm not happy with, then I can remind them this should be done, this should be followed up, write it in their notes. If I'm concerned about it, I speak to [the team leader], where it's her position to do anything further.

While Karen has a designated clinical supervision role, she perceives that her position is only to *advise* healthworkers. In her view, it is the team leader's responsibility, as the line manager, to formally direct healthworkers.

Clinical priorities versus client priorities

In similar fashion to other AHS nurses, Karen suggests that in comparison to a healthworker, a nursing background gives her better diagnostic and curative skills, more specific knowledge of medications and their effects, and more understanding of the progression of illness and disease. In contrast to the nursing role, Karen describes the healthworker as a 'health visitor' with both clinical monitoring and welfare duties:

> Their main role now is a health visitor—for checking their blood pressure, blood sugar, making sure their medications are all up to date and doing the welfare side of things, which is always there for everyone in [the AHS] … Forty per cent upwards of your work is welfare, family business.

While Karen emphasises clinical monitoring and views welfare tasks as an additional component of healthworker practice, Jeanne, her predecessor, emphasises its holistic scope and recognises that health-workers inevitably fail to fully complete all tasks:

> When caring for someone, you don't just look at health needs, there's also welfare … and emotional needs. You spend time—if someone is out of household gas, you look at that. Whereas the Community Nursing Agency can go in, dress the dressing and the job's done. Part of holistic is education as well—that's important, but you haven't got time to sit down and address it 'cause there is so much else impacting on one's time. So in the end, you're a jack of all trades and master of none.

Karen suggests that while healthworkers deal well with welfare problems, their clinical skills are weak, and may not even be valued by clients:

> The welfare stuff works well. There's always a back up, there's always someone to talk about problems with your bills and your housing and your Housing Commission problems and all that—that stuff works really well … But just the medical health side of things, it could improve a lot … I don't think they are functioning effectively as *health* workers in my view … If we're going to be a *health* worker in terms of looking at people's health and illnesses, you either do

that or forget that whole side and just provide care-aides, social care, which is what a lot of the clients want more than the healthworker visits. They want all that other stuff—they're not particularly interested in having their [clinical] bits and pieces done.

As do doctors and other AHS nurses, both Jeanne, here, and Karen observe that healthworkers underestimate the significance of clinical indicators:

Clinical skills need to be upgraded as well, and put into proper perspective … It's like you get this knowledge—their training showed them blood sugar levels, blood pressure and taking weight. It was one thing to do it, something else to know what to do *with* it.

Karen suggests that the designation *health* worker, along with Family Care's claim to provide medical care, demand the delivery of competent clinical services. Two factors thwart such delivery: healthworkers are not sufficiently competent clinicians, and, incongruously, many chronically ill clients give priority to social problems:

All the [welfare] sort of stuff that needs to be sorted out as a priority, they'll want to get all that sorted out. Often you'll have to deal with all that stuff before you can look at the gammy leg, gangrenous toe or whatever—sort all that out first, and then we can look at some of the health issues later, when you are a bit more calm and relaxed about things.

This recognition that many clients accord personal health concerns less priority than their social problems echoes Rita and Merle in Chapter 2. Consequently, Karen emphasises the task of making clinical health a priority for clients.

'Working in closely'

Karen suggests that healthworkers should advocate the importance of health to their frail and aged clients:

I often see that as a healthworker our goal should be, try to make their health a priority for them. Because they're not gonna make it a priority, so it's almost like taking over that role. 'We'll look after that side for you 'cause we know you're not going to—make sure you get your regular checks, make sure you're keeping everything down within the safety zone so you're not going to have a heart attack or have a stroke or drop over'.

Whereas doctors expect a client referral, Karen advocates that if healthworkers record abnormal clinical readings consistently, they should 'work in closely with the client':

If it's just a one-off, you accept that as a one-off. But if it's repeated, something needs to be done because something is definitely very wrong—either working in with them really closely to monitor it, you either pick up your visits, increase your visits to monitor them a bit more closely and get a clearer picture of what's going on. If you're not sure if they're taking their medicine, try and get quite close in on that to see if, maybe, they're just not taking their tablets, or maybe they've got so many tablets they're getting confused and they should really have a dossette box. Just say, 'Alright, we're going to put your tablets in a dossette box'.

Jeanne advocates a similar approach:

If it's never been picked up by a doctor, they should be taken to the doctor. If they are already on medication, if they are established on medication, they should be asked about their diet, their exercise and their stress level. [The healthworker] needs to sit down and say, 'How can we undertake some of these things?' 'They've got to sit down and educate them … get a routine where we walk to the shop, and chat to them and educate them on the way.

Karen, indicates that this approach can have dramatic positive effects:

Jennifer, poor love, she has high blood pressure, she used to be shocking. Now, since she's got a dossette box that gets filled every week, she's incredible. She used to be coming into the clinic every couple of weeks with [urinary tract infections], her urine was full of sugar. So that's just been something really simple which has really improved her health, heaps.

If nothing changes after 'working in closely', the field nurses expect the healthworker to organise a clinical consultation and to follow up with the doctor. Karen emphasises continuity of care: the need for healthworkers to follow up with both the doctor and the client:

So once you've worked in closely with that, and you know that everything is being done that should be done and there's no change, then that's when they need to be seen by the doctor. So to organise that they get seen by the doctor ... or get the client to make an appointment—either way, it doesn't matter so long as they get to see someone. And any other sort of follow-up on that—see what the doctor does, speak to the doctor, find out any changes, treatment regime, follow that through.

Hindrances to continuity of care

Like the AHS doctors, both Karen and Jeanne perceive that many healthworkers fail to maintain follow-up. According to Jeanne:

Initially they were visiting and just recording. Initially it was so hard getting into this pattern of working, recording what you'd done, following up what you're doing ... You've got to remember I was a nurse as well. I was pretty pedantic about things like that— for example, recording what you had done and follow-ups. I was trained under the old system, which was task oriented.

Karen also reports difficulties ensuring that healthworkers monitor client progress and do the necessary follow-ups, and she attributes these difficulties to cultural traits. To encourage them to follow up, Karen provides reminders:

> I will write notes pointing out the things that need to be done, specialist appointments to be done, and I'll come back a few months later and none of it's been done. I've spoken to them about it, but 'Oh' she said, 'I've moved on to the next section [in the file]' …
>
> It's really hard, whole different concepts of care y'know, like the idea of continual care or following through care. They all live day to day. Life for a blackfella is day to day, and that really flows into their work, so they look at what that is today. It's really hard to be looking at things over time and seeing them recurring over time, to actually look back through their file, go back to look at what's been happening, to see the picture.

Not only does 'culture' explain the lack of follow-up but, according to Karen, it also fosters an acceptance of illness and disease:

> It's a culture of acceptance of illness and sickness and death as being just something that happens and really can't be prevented. You can see how all the healthworkers here, all the Aboriginal staff here, how often they have to go to funerals. It's unreal how many funerals they attend. A whitefella wouldn't attend that many in a lifetime. For anyone who's twenty-five, Aboriginal, that age, they've been to so many funerals, that's just life doing its thing … Maybe it's blackfella way to, y'know, just to accept life's processes a lot more as well.

However, Jeanne, the Aboriginal field nurse, suggests that the nature of the social context hinders follow-up: both healthworkers and clients become embroiled in immediate needs arising from persistent social problems:

> The healthworkers themselves got too caught up in the felt needs themselves, they couldn't stand back from it … The healthworkers

were not objective—you work here and you react to everyday goings on. People's attitudes have an impact on you, it distorts clear goals, you are continually having to react to the now. The now is important to Aboriginal people. It's too difficult to stand back and plan—we had good focus, but they get distracted, it's everyday things that gets in the way. When you're in the thick of it you have to respond, you can't walk away. The healthworkers haven't been trained in that …

You come in the office to start your day, you've got your plan—you'll go visit Myrtle or granny, whoever. And the telephone rings, you take the call, 'Why blah blah blah????' You immediately get caught, it puts your day out of kilter, it can make you angry. The management of that is hard … for example, a death could happen. The person you've planned to be with, they'll get upset, they expect you to be there. It's like the healthworkers are in constant turmoil—there's nothing clear-cut with Aboriginal things.

In order to survive constant exposure to 'turmoil', Jeanne suggests that healthworkers need sophisticated negotiation skills, ways to respond appropriately—to say, 'I realise you've got a problem now—I've made other commitments, I'll get back to you'.

In short, Jeanne observes that when healthworkers are 'in the thick of it', they lack the capacity to negotiate skilfully. As a result, they are in 'constant turmoil', unable to maintain a clinical focus or to make clinical health a priority for clients.

The need for professional relationships

Karen suggests that healthworker relationships with clients are counterproductive, and observes that their communication is insufficiently health oriented. She identifies a 'cultural' orientation, with healthworkers treating abnormal clinical readings too lightly:

I've been out with them. It's like a joke's made about it a bit—'Oh that's a bit high!' They'll have a laugh about it, which is fine if it's a one-off thing, but … it seems like the culture of the organisation. It's really hard to be serious about what you're doing.

In contrast, Karen advocates the delivery of clear and straightforward advice to clients:

> Like if you have a big heart-to-heart with the client about: 'If your blood pressure is going to stay like this you are going to have a stroke, there is no doubt about it—we've got to work really hard on getting this down, otherwise you're going to be dead'. Or your blood sugar, or you're going to be blind, or you're going to be on dialysis in a couple of years.

Karen describes a client who has not received the appropriate messages about her problems. She despairs that a tragic outcome is imminent:

> Annie is a classic. She's only a young woman, she's only in her forties. I've been seeing that picture where Annie's sugar's just really bad for many years ... normal is between 4 and 8, hers would commonly be in the high teens or 20s. I mean, she doesn't even have a blood sugar machine to check her own sugars ... She's been on our programme for years ... You really need to work in closely with someone like that, encouraging them to have annual checks. That should be arranged by the healthworkers, so the specialist can actually pick up any problems that are starting early, just preventive y'know. She's probably going to be on dialysis before Christmas ... that's if she doesn't die before then, and she's only in her forties. You see these things happening, you open the files and look at them and I can see just what's happened. I can see the stroke that was coming or I can see the laser treatment for the eyes—there's a reason why.

Rather than their relationships with clients being serious and professional, Karen observes that for most healthworkers they are more like a friendship:

Theirs becomes very much a friendship, very much a friendship ... that's the way they relate, very open hearted and jovial ... always trying to make each other feel better—always trying to make each other feel better and lighten the awful things that are happening to their bodies, to their friends, to their community.

Paradoxically, while Karen questions this provision of emotional support, a welfare worker quoted above describes this facet of health-worker practice as an asset. For Karen, it hinders clinical practice. Her conversations with clients result in the acquisition of crucial health information, which she considers is due partly to her status as a nurse. She notes that clients don't even expect such questions from healthworkers:

When I go out with the girls, sometimes we'll come away and they'll say, 'How did you get all that information out of them? They've never talked to me about that.' So some of them won't talk to the healthworkers about some things ... my relationship with them is different, and they'll talk to me about medical things—they see me as sister/nurse ... That's the client's perception of healthworkers, y'know, they don't expect that from these health-workers.

To a degree, Karen's observations of client expectations match healthworker feedback reported in Chapter 2: clients do not see some interventions as within the healthworker role. Nevertheless, like some AHS doctors, Karen judges that healthworkers lack the ability to probe deeply into client health problems. In contrast, she considers herself to be somewhat of a 'busybody':

They don't know how to ask the questions to get that informa-tion—to probe and chat and to find out more things about what's going on. You have to be really inquisitive, you have to be a real busybody, really ... they all tell me information and things about themselves that even the healthworkers say, 'I never knew that'. But I go and talk about health things with them—whether it's their bladder, if they've got troubles with their bladder or their eyesight, how they're managing moving around the house … which I think the healthworkers feel embarrassed about.

Rather than risking embarrassment through talking about 'health things', Karen proposes that healthworkers take a more social orientation:

All the conversation that goes with healthworkers' work is social conversation. They're the networks for them to find out how's whatsy doing, who died and what's happening there.

In brief, both Karen and Jeanne indicate that a variety of factors inhibit the capacity of healthworkers to manage clients' clinical conditions. These factors include: 1) a social context that induces both clients and healthworkers to focus mainly on social rather than clinical needs; 2) a lack of clinical understandings among healthworkers that results in inaction over abnormal clinical readings; 3) an informal healthworker/ client relationship that leaves healthworkers relatively uninformed about clinical problems.

Karen suggests that healthworkers engage informally not only with clients, but also with her as their supervisor. She finds clinical supervision easier in a less formal situation. Previously, her desk sat in the same large room as the healthworkers, and she could review their work informally. Now in a separate office, she reports that both she and the healthworkers experience considerable discomfort during supervision. Karen observes that when healthworkers need to debrief, they prefer to do so informally amongst themselves:

They all unload with each other—they all have each other, the healthworkers … A lot of the time is spent sitting out the front having a fag and having cups of tea—that might go on for hours, all that … Although they will talk about the need to have more, the opportunity to offload and discuss things … but when that happens it's often hard. You get a formal situation, it won't work.

As with their more informal relationships with clients, Karen indicates that in relation to both the technical and emotional components of clinical supervision, healthworkers prefer more informal processes. She observes that this is also true of training.

Incomplete training

Both Karen and Jeanne judge that healthworker training is incomplete, and Karen's response is to provide more training herself. Jeanne thinks the training is too theoretical:

> My expectation of them was to be self-directed. The initial healthworker course didn't allow for that. There was too much theory and not enough practice. The potential was there but it needed development … there was a gap between the knowledge and actually applying it in the situation.

Karen observes that the training focuses more on 'wellness' rather on than curative care:

> I know the healthworker training is more of wellness-related type approach and a wellness model … but so many people are sick, that's the fact of it, and you need to know how to treat people who are ill, 'cause you are not going to be coming into contact with many people who are well.

Because morbidity is so high, Karen advocates a strong emphasis on clinical skills and curative care. Like the doctors, she points to a need for healthworkers to specialise, and to be trained in that specialisation. However, she recognises that the diverse needs of clients make it difficult to designate a particular specialisation:

> I mean, there is so much stuff that healthworkers have to be taught, that they wanted to teach them, and it's really hard to know what area to focus in. I mean, every area is such a specialty, has to be a

specialty area. They could have done all their training just in aged care, diabetes … they could have done three years to be working here, but they've had a whole lot of training in other areas as well.

In summary, the nurses who supervise and monitor day-to-day healthworker practice clearly recognise both the clinical ailments and the persistent social disruptions that impact upon client lives. The Family Care field nurses acknowledge that clients place priority on resolving social problems and that healthworkers respond to these competently. Nevertheless, there is also a suggestion that, because they lack appropriate negotiation and bargaining skills, healthworkers can get caught up and thrown into turmoil by client social problems, to the detriment of a clinical focus and subsequent follow-up. This tendency, the nurses observe, is fostered by insufficient specific clinical training, particularly of practical skills learned hands-on, and by the informal style of relationship preferred by healthworkers. They advocate that healthworkers should work in closely with clients to ensure that health becomes the client's priority.

CLIENT AND COLLEAGUE PERSPECTIVES OVERALL

Most stakeholders in the activities of Family Care healthworkers observe them from a considerable distance, and inevitably this leads to some misunderstandings. Confusion about the role of healthworkers is exacerbated by a number of factors: 1) according to the nurses, confusion results from misleading and inaccurate understandings about the healthworker role being promoted by senior managers and bureaucrats; 2) in the case of support staff, misunderstandings result from a lack of in-house professional orientation to the purpose and scope of the healthworker practice; and 3) in the case of doctors, there is an absence of clear communication channels and supervision structures enabling clinical review to inform field work, and vice-versa. Thus the nature of healthworker practice remains open to speculation, assumptions and rumour.

Nevertheless, the clinical knowledge and skills of healthworkers are a major concern for both doctors and nurses. While clients express appreciation both of regular clinical monitoring and of healthworkers maintaining an overview of their health, doctors and nurses remain sceptical. In their view, the lack of response by healthworkers to abnormal clinical indicators indicates that their clinical understandings and skills are inadequate. Nurses feel that in comparison, their training gives them far better diagnostic and curative skills, more specific knowledge of medications and more understanding of the progression of disease and illness. As a result, nurses oppose positioning healthworkers as the first point of contact with clients.

Doctors and nurses also view follow-up by healthworkers as a problem. Because doctors conclude that clients are unlikely to attend to their own health problems, they propose that healthworkers should follow up in order to reinforce the message, and they suggest more frequent follow-up with AHS doctors and local GPs. The Aboriginal field nurse observes that because of the demands of the 'now', the healthworkers are in 'constant turmoil' and become over-extended, which explains, in part, their lack of attention to clinical monitoring and follow-up.

She views their practice as holistic and gives equal emphasis to their clinical and social interventions. In her view, healthworkers often lack adequate negotiation skills to deal with the chaotic context of Aboriginal community life, and therefore fall into the role of a Jack of all trades. A Welfare worker also observes the 'turmoil' of healthworkers and the stress of their working environment. Both he and the field nurses recognise a crucial need for healthworkers to debrief.

The communication skills of the healthworkers and their relationships with clients are also criticised by some doctors and nurses. While clients report that it feels good to be seen by an Aboriginal person, both doctors and nurses question the ability of healthworkers to ask clients strategic health-related questions. The non-Aboriginal field nurse perceives that healthworkers have not so much a professional relationship as an informal friendship with clients, focused on social and emotional support. Paradoxically, other workers view this as an asset.

Doctors and nurses propose improved healthworker training. Most nurses consider that healthworkers require a more systemic understanding of the body in order to interpret clinical data. Doctors and nurses advocate more practical training in a structured and super-vised environment, and more exposure to the training of other health professionals. Doctors recommend greater emphasis on inter-personal investigative skills and on the understanding of medications and the effects of polypharmacy. Both doctors and nurses suggest that health-workers need depth of training in specific areas rather than training as broad generalists. Doctors also suggest specialised in-service training, ongoing refresher courses and practical supervision.

In general terms, the common view among their colleagues that healthworkers could do more to assist them reflects a perception of plasticity in healthworker practice. While they all regard healthworkers as potential assistants, there is no clear consensus about what should be the focus of their work. The only consensus centres on a clinical orien-tation to curative care rather than a client-centred, holistic, preventive casework practice. This orientation resonates with clinical health professionals, their current training, understandings and perceptions of need. The emphasis on clinical monitoring and care does not, however, speak to the chaotic social and cultural disruption experienced daily by healthworkers delivering services beyond the clinic.

These perceptions of their colleagues stand in marked contrast to healthworkers' own perceptions of their work. Healthworkers express a need for greater support and recognition for their client-centred holistic practice, in order to deal effectively with the complex situations faced by their clients. Their perception of a lack of professional recognition and support is the focus of the next chapter.

CHAPTER — 4

Engaging the Health System

Many assertions have been made about the importance of Aboriginal healthworkers within Aboriginal health policy, but their place within the health system has not been clearly articulated. They work in an organisational borderland, with indeterminate status and no clear boundaries. Their professional colleagues rarely grant them serious recognition as fellow professionals, and their practice is often contingent upon decisions of nurses and doctors. Even the respect accorded them by their clients is variable. Due to their marginal status, they are highly vulnerable to exploitation.

LACK OF IDENTITY, VOICE AND STATUS

'We don't get enough say'

The healthworkers express concerns about their lack of professional recognition and status within both the Aboriginal Health Service and the wider health arena. In particular, they seek more recognition for their distinct professional practice and greater involvement in the planning and co-ordination of services.

Ruby has had seven years of experience as a Family Care healthworker. She completed twelve years of schooling and has obtained both a healthworker certificate and a university degree in Indigenous community health. Having the necessary educational credentials, she co-ordinates her own programme and expects to make a difference. However, she finds her practice is consistently subjected to the priorities of others. This book begins with Ruby's words, which are repeated and expanded here.

Following a particularly frustrating staff meeting, she sits with her colleague Merle at the kitchen table in the staffroom. Gloomily resting her cheek in her cupped hand, she broods pessimistically on the potential of healthworkers to change the status of Aboriginal health:

> They wanted all us healthworkers 'cause we were going to change everything, but we're so strictly dictated to, it's changed nothing. Some of us have great ideas, and we could do it all, but we just can't do it. Instead of like handing things to us, we're always dictated to … we don't get enough say in the programme … I thought yes, we've got a power, we're united, but then last week it just killed it … We say we want to have our own voice, [but] you should've been there—there was all these powerful healthworkers that just agreed to everything [the nurse] said … People are still dying—Teddy's going to get his toes cut off, Daisy died … people are just dying of things that could have been changed. I mean, they may just as well employ community nurses.

Ruby's anguished recognition is that neither she nor her colleagues have sufficient authority to make a significant impact. Despite claims about the central role of Aboriginal healthworkers, Ruby finds that they are unable to effect any notable changes. In her view, this is because other health professionals control their work. She sees that her own people are needlessly suffering and dying, that healthworkers have few opportunities to make change individually, that they have limited collective power and lack collective confidence. Labouring under the 'dictates' of other professionals, Ruby suggests that healthworkers are unable to provide a service distinct from that of the community nurses. Consequently, she concludes that healthworkers lack any discernible professional identity.

Ruby's words capture both her frustration and her pain. Just as her clients exist on the fringe of the mainstream health system, Ruby suggests that so do the healthworkers, even those within Aboriginal community-controlled health organisations.

'We're always dictated to'

According to Ruby, Aboriginal Health Service doctors, who stress biomedical interventions, play a major role in the formulation of client care plans. In her view, healthworkers differ from doctors in terms of the nature of services required by clients. Ruby observes that health-workers subscribe to a more holistic model of health, focused on client need. She describes a healthworker:

> Someone who can do more than one thing. They're not just trained in paramedical, they've got skills in counselling … We do many things—you can't say we just do that one thing … getting food for people, funerals, getting brothers and sisters together … getting families together, mediating a lot of family argument … [This work happens] mostly in their houses, but we do a lot of follow-up at the medical service—ringing welfare agencies, making appointments, contacting other family members, writing all the letters … lots and lots of things to do. Things don't stop out here [in the field] unfortunately.

Rita too suggests that a healthworker is a practitioner of a client-centred holistic approach to health care. During a Family Care staff meeting the team leader, Rose, identifies the principal aim of the Family Care section: 'It's providing holistic care … to our frail-aged and younger disabled'.

However, Ruby observes that a holistic approach often conflicts with the clinical monitoring that doctors perceive as their most important task. In particular, she expresses frustration with doctors who blame her and her colleagues for failing to monitor client medications, especially in situations where they are responding to conflicting but equally essential needs, such as obtaining food supplies:

We had a meeting with the medical people, when I was in [the Family Care programme]. I said, 'Well if I go to someone's house and they don't want their BSL [blood sugar level] or BP [blood pressure] checked, and they would rather I take them shopping', I said, 'Alright then, that's what I'll do'. But [the doctors] said, 'No, you should make them have their BP and BSL done—that's what you're employed to do'.

Despite the doctors' views, Ruby is adamant that a wider focus is necessary to meet the expressed needs of clients:

We've got to focus our service on the client and what the client wants. I mean, it would be lovely if I just went to see [a client], do a blood pressure—and come back in. That meets the service guidelines, but [it] doesn't meet the client's needs.

Ruby suggests that most doctors lack sufficient understanding of the context of Aboriginal people's lives to appreciate the potential for a broad role to make tangible improvement. While acknowledging that the community nurses also work in the field, Ruby thinks that their narrower biomedical focus confines them to a limited view of the client's world.

In brief, Ruby proposes that a holistic health practice includes the social, emotional and spiritual wellbeing of clients. In her experience, doctors and nurses often ignore these vitally important aspects of Aboriginal health. Ruby's distress at the ignorance of some doctors is made evident in a presentation to the Second National Aboriginal and Torres Strait Islander Health Worker Conference:

My story relates more to frustrations with other health professionals and how they treat the healthworker role. My story relates to a lady who was on the Family Care programme for about four weeks. I actually went to visit the lady in her home. When I got there, there was no family at home and she told me that she was dying and she wanted to die at home. I asked her whether she wanted me to call an ambulance or something like that. She said no, she just wanted to be left at home; so, I said I would go and call an AHS doctor—just to make sure she was comfortable and that there was nothing else we could do. Because she had no phone at her house, I had to go down the road to use the public phone.

The AHS doctor rang an ambulance and the lady was taken to hospital before I got back to the house. She later died in hospital. The family was informed by the police.

When I got back to the AHS, they told me not to worry about it because I had done all that a healthworker could do. I was left very frustrated that they didn't respect my healthworker role with the client—and that they thought that my decision wasn't good enough—and that the doctor had the right, and the nurse had the right, to over-rule my decision.

Ruby's experience suggests a significant lack of respect and regard not only for her Indigenous cultural values (which place high importance on family presence at the time of death) and her professional competence, but also for the integrity of her unique relationship with the client.

A further frustration for healthworkers is the failure of some doctors to acknowledge their schedule of duties. Healthworkers service a client caseload requiring daily home visits. Because they have commitments in the field, the healthworkers find demands of doctors unrealistic:

Merle: See, I don't think the doctors realise, like when they ring up and they want us over there, they don't realise that we might be just going out to see clients. When they ring, they want you there …

Rita: No, they're [very] rude.

Ruby: [A doctor] did that to me the other day.

Rita: They upset me.

Merle: And the thing is …

Rita: And they think that you're goin' to run around for them, and drive here and drive there, when you need to go and see [other clients].

Disparate views towards healthworker practice create communication difficulties, confusion and conflict. Healthworkers claim that doctors frequently fail to consult them, blame them unfairly for not monitoring a client's condition and, in response to client complaints, listen only to the client's story. The tension between healthworkers and doctors also characterises their relationships with nurses.

Notwithstanding the views of the other health professionals in the organisation, Ruby maintains that healthworkers have a role beyond a narrow clinical approach. Further, she perceives that unlike periodic biomedical monitoring, a client-centred holistic practice provides tangible, positive health outcomes:

> I can see the difference it makes to offer people extra home help—not as much paramedical—and to buy supplies for everyone, cotton and things, and to help—not to offer just a physical visiting service ... What extra we do is what keeps them in the house ... I mean you can go once a week and you can do blood pressures, you can do sugar levels, you can make sure they've got tablets—nothing is ever going to improve, there's really no point in going there ... what have you changed?

According to Ruby, not only is a narrow clinical monitoring role (servicing 'paramedical' needs) of limited benefit, but as the sole focus of work, it is detrimental to healthworker effectiveness. She claims that the pressure to follow a narrow clinical approach inhibits the initiative and confidence of healthworkers to engage, for example, in teaching clients how to self-manage their health or in advocacy work to prevent client evictions.

The case of Teddy

The holistic practice of healthworkers is unrecognised not only in their own organisation, but also in health contexts outside the AHS. Client advocacy and support during external consultations with mainstream service providers is an important component of Family Care healthworker services. Yet Ruby experiences a lack of recognition for her qualifications, experience and skills in this area. The case of Teddy, outlined at the start of Chapter 1, is a graphic example.

Teddy is a young client who suffers disabilities as a result of non-insulin-dependent diabetes. He is visited daily by a healthworker, who monitors his blood sugar level and blood pressure, changes his dressings and advocates for him to other health and welfare professionals. After a hospital admission, Merle attempts to visit him, but finds he has already been discharged. Later that day she visits him at home and, upon applying fresh dressings to his feet, she finds maggots in the wound. When Ruby challenges the nursing staff at both the District and the General hospitals, they disbelieve and dismiss her complaints. This case shows how a lack of professional recognition by other health professionals compromises healthworker effectiveness.

Ruby sees that this lack of recognition and respect undermines healthworker confidence and, ultimately, professional morale and identity. She experiences disrespect not only in personal interaction, but also through the organisational structures of the AHS—where she claims healthworkers have little say in programme planning or decision-making.

'We have great ideas'

In Ruby's perception, although healthworkers have significant practical knowledge to contribute to the development of programmes and policy, invitations to be genuine participants in planning are rare:

> When they set up teams to work on programme development, there are very few healthworkers—or healthworkers that work in the field … [The] doctors who see the clients in the clinic, they don't know what's happening out in the community. I can't see how they can develop programmes that are going to work in the community without the knowledge of people who work in that area. What does it say for us? That we're *just* delivering the service—and we don't get a say in how it's run—or whether it's going to work or not.

She suggests that healthworkers, despite their unique understanding of client needs, have marginal input into the development of community outreach programmes. In particular, she proposes that their qualifications and field experience provide healthworkers with the necessary credentials to judge the appropriateness of such programmes. For example, she believes that the environmental health standards of nurses and doctors may be inappropriate to the reality of the task.

Ruby relates the case of a nurse who visited a Family Care client. Upon her return to the clinic, the nurse reported to the doctor that the client's house was uncharacteristically filthy. The doctor 'demanded' an explanation. Ruby informed the doctor that the disabled client cleaned the house herself and mopped her own floors. Although the floors were not generally 'sparkling' clean, they were hygienic, and the client was proud of her own efforts.

While the doctor criticised Ruby for allowing the client to live in such circumstances, Ruby felt that compared with both this particular client's previous history and with other clients, the house was satisfactory. In making her evaluation, Ruby considered crucial contextual issues including the client's self-esteem and the need to maintain an effective relationship. According to criteria to which the doctor is oblivious, Ruby judged the house acceptable.

Ruby perceives that both doctors and nurses plan and develop policy and programmes without adequate understanding either of the community context or of the healthworker's role. She claims that lack of acknowledgement of healthworkers, despite their qualifications, and their lack of 'say' in policy and programme development, results in healthworkers seeking alternative work:

> People that are healthworkers at the medical service don't work as healthworkers ... the person who works in the dentist, she's a healthworker; one of the receptionists was a healthworker for a long time; one of the transport drivers, he's a healthworker ...

She and her colleagues advocate that healthworkers, alongside doctors as consultants on biomedical needs, have a central role in the co-ordination of client care. They suggest such an approach in relation to a new programme that uses healthworkers to provide outreach services to families:

> **Rose**: The thing is, if we allow the doctors to have too much say in their care plan, it is all going to be too medically orientated … And we need to back away from that … because the client is going to agree to whatever the doctor says. They're not going to say, 'No I don't agree with that'. The doctor will say, 'What about we do this, this and this', and they're going to sit there and say, 'Yes, yes, yes'. Because then the doctor is the main actor. They're not going to say, 'I don't agree with that, I don't want that' … The healthworker should be there, so the health-worker can say to the client, 'Look, you don't have to agree with this if you don't want to, if you feel there's no need to change'.
>
> **Ruby**: I disagree with doctors doing care plans.
>
> **Rita**: So do I—especially with Aboriginal people.
>
> **June**: Yep, Yep.
>
> **Ruby**: My argument then is, why should the doctor write up the thing? Someone who knows Daisy like me or a healthworker, who's worked with Daisy, they should draw up that care plan—like go and talk to the doctor about what are her biomedical needs.
>
> **Rita**: 'Cause I think the healthworker has to be the key role for it to work.
>
> **Ruby**: Or someone who is not medically orientated.
>
> **Rita**: A healthworker …
>
> **June**: If they don't do it off on the blackfella's basis, the blackfella's grassroots level, it's not going to work at all.

Healthworkers stress familiarity with the community context as the necessary basis for the co-ordination of client care. However, the usual experience for healthworkers is that other health professionals determine the directions of their work.

In short, Ruby's experience is that healthworkers have little say in health planning within the AHS. She suggests that they are both marginal to the agendas and subject to the 'dictates' of doctors and nurses. In her view, this occurs despite healthworkers' qualifications, their unique Indigenous knowledge and their significant experience in administering practical day-to-day care in the community. Her conclusion is that rather than play a central role in Aboriginal health, healthworkers 'just deliver a service'.

The case of Daisy

The case of Ruby's client Daisy reveals the challenges to healthworker morale and efficacy that result from a lack of voice in the provision of care. The following account draws directly on my observations of Ruby's relationship with her client.

Out on a home visit, Ruby pulls up outside a double-fronted, 1960s era, cream brick-veneer house in the suburbs. A V8 Holden Commodore, a Ford station wagon, a powerboat on a trailer and an older sedan car all sit embedded in the sand patch that extends to the street front. Ruby calls out 'Hello', and enters the open door leading into the front room of the house. A young woman welcomes her. Three mop-haired children come bursting into the room, scragging each other. The front room has a low ceiling and is grey and spare. Vinyl tiles cover the concrete floor. Large posters and an Aboriginal flag cover one wall. Underneath the flag is a vinyl settee with raw foam cushions. In the corner, a person lies in an iron hospital bed tilted up at the head. To the side, on an intravenous infusion stand, hangs a limp saline bag and tube. Further to the right, a veneer and glass sideboard is covered with medical wrappers, pills and paraphernalia, in the midst of which sits a white rectangular box hand-labelled in blue biro, 'For Runs'. A few flies circle in the half-light from the curtained windows. Suddenly the wrestling turns to tears as a child howls at the young woman's knee, an event apparently unnoticed by the figure in the bed.

The person in the bed is a slight, wiry, fuzzy-haired Aboriginal woman of perhaps sixty years. She appears to be dozing. Ruby says hello to her, and a smile breaks across her face. Ruby's client is on home dialysis for renal failure. She recently suffered a heart attack and has diabetes with peripheral neuropathy in her feet. Ruby removes the covers from Daisy's feet, and her toes protrude above the bed-end. They are swollen and raw. Two toes are missing. According to Ruby, her feet may require further amputation. She is suffering from severe bedsores. Four days earlier, Daisy visited the podiatrist and the doctor at the AHS. Both decided she needed to be in hospital. Admitted on the Friday, the hospital discharged her on Sunday. Prior to admission, Ruby informed Daisy that the hospital would look after her for a couple of weeks until her foot healed.

Ruby examines her foot. The skin graft over the amputated toe is turning black. The next toe is also black and gangrenous. Daisy has a large ulcer on her anklebone. She is in pain, and cries out as Ruby examines her foot. Ruby then goes outside to telephone the AHS. Daisy asks for assistance to turn on her side. Her husband supports her shoulders and turns her around, and Daisy cries out again. Ruby returns and has a brief conversation with the husband and daughter, informing them that Daisy needs hospital care. She tells the family that an AHS doctor will ring the hospital and organise for her admission. When Daisy is informed, she is unwilling to go to hospital. 'Do you wanna get your leg cut off?' queries her husband.

Driving back to the AHS, Ruby says that the worst thing about the situation is that now she has to go and 'argue' Daisy's case with the doctors. Upon her return, Ruby talks to the Family Care field nurse, who in turn talks to the doctor. The nurse later informs Ruby that Daisy can possibly go into the extended care section of the General Hospital.

The next morning I ask Ruby, 'Is she in hospital?' Obviously distressed, Ruby replies, 'No', and looks away. Moments later her care-aide in the Chronic Care programme, Monica, returns from visiting Daisy and reports that she is not at home because the family have taken her to hospital.

A week later Ruby informs me that Daisy has septicaemia and a staphylococcus infection in the toe. She is not responding to medica-tion. The anaesthetist cannot risk 'putting her under' for the operation on the foot. Ruby appears disheartened and morose. She is concerned she will be blamed for Daisy's condition. Her opinion is that 'blood poisoning is preventable; it could have been prevented'.

In the office on the following Monday morning, the care-aide informs me that Daisy died the previous Friday. Ruby's response suggests a range of emotions. She appears both frustrated and upset at her inability to ensure the necessary care for Daisy. She seems astonished that the hospital discharged Daisy three times, with no apparent concern for the gangrene. She says she feels that she has 'failed'. And she is grieving the loss of a person with whom she has established a long and close relationship.

The death of clients is not uncommon for healthworkers. In fact, the presence of death is a frequent experience in their work. In a grief counselling workshop offered to healthworkers, Ruby shares her feelings about becoming 'cold' to the deaths of clients:

> When people die a lot, you soon get cold to it. I don't like to say it, but that's how it is. The first couple you love, you feel it, then you get numb … So—you just get used to it, people dying, clients just die, you get cold. I could go to a family's funeral, and it would be like it didn't matter.

Merle, like the other healthworkers, shares Ruby's constant exposure to death: 'You read about it you know, but it doesn't really hit you until you're [working in the AHS]. All the deaths, all the deaths—I can't get over it.' And Josie says, 'I've been working here for nearly five years and I have never been to so many funerals'.

It is clear that through their regular home visits, healthworkers become part of the daily rhythm of their clients' lives. They spend time sitting in kitchens, talking with family members, sharing community news, walking around the block, going to professional appointments, sharing joys, pains and heartaches. They give support when clients are dying, then deal with the deep feelings that arise when death puts an end to close relationships with clients and their families. Christine, a colleague of Ruby's, shares the depth of her own experience:

The day he passed away, it was just like part of my world [disappeared]—it's like that with all our oldies. That's why I think we should have a lot more counselling. It takes a hell of a lot out of you … they really start to depend on you in the end … With a lot of our oldies that are passing away, people think that once they're dead that's it—they don't realise the grieving we go through too.

In brief, the death of clients or their carers is a common occurrence for the healthworkers. In attempting to ensure access and care for their clients, healthworkers have minimal authority and are dependent on the judgements of other health professionals. Ruby's frustration is that her assessment of Daisy's condition has no standing. She has no power to change anything, yet she is left nursing the consequences. Rather than playing a pivotal role in Aboriginal health, Ruby suggests that people die from 'things that could have been changed' and, overall, healthworkers have 'changed nothing'.

'Healthworkers were going to change everything …'

Ruby qualifies as an Aboriginal healthworker on two counts: 1) she is Indigenous, and it is recognised that her life experience gives her a unique understanding of the wellbeing of her own people; 2) she has an accredited healthworker qualification. Drawing upon her own experience and training, and in accordance with the prevailing service delivery philosophy of her workplace, she practises and advocates a client-centred holistic approach to meeting the health needs of Aboriginal clients. From this viewpoint, health encompasses not only the physical wellbeing of clients, but also their particular social, cultural, emotional and spiritual needs.

The client-centred holistic approach makes sense to Ruby. It recognises the prevalence of a wide range of health determinants amongst her clients. Many of these are social determinants, such as inadequate housing. Ruby finds that by reducing the impact of these factors on the lives of her frail-aged and elderly clients, their health improves: 'We have to focus our service on the client … what extra we do … is what prevents them going into a nursing home or getting evicted'.

Ruby and her healthworker colleagues observe that other health professionals and managers disregard or dismiss their Aboriginality, training, qualifications, unique practice and experience. Yet they believe that potentially they have a central role to play in the development of community health services for Aboriginal clients.

CLAIMING A PROFESSIONAL DOMAIN

A perceived lack of professional recognition prompted the healthworkers to engage in collective action. Their complaints at the lack of professional recognition by nurses, and grievances by nurses about the scope of healthworker activities, eventually provoked an organisational response. Three forums convened within the AHS provided healthworkers with the opportunity to articulate their concerns. The forums included a combined workshop of healthworkers and nurses to distinguish their respective roles, a workshop for healthworkers focusing on strategies to enhance their organisational status, and a series of meetings of a small healthworker association within the AHS, the Indigenous Healthworker Coalition.

The bottom-up and the top-down

A planning meeting prior to the combined workshop for healthworkers and nurses enabled the healthworkers to clarify their concerns. Josie reports that while collecting medications from the clinic, the clinic sister had interrogated her about drugs and their dosages: 'she was treating me like I didn't know what I was on about'. On another occasion, after reviewing an elderly client at the request of a nurse, Josie requested the nurse to examine a client's children. She reports that she received no response. Rita claims that having received permission to weigh a client using the clinic scales, the same nurse subsequently reprimanded her for using them.

The healthworkers all say they feel 'looked down upon' by nurses. Ruby observes that nurses hold a different understanding of health service delivery: that whereas healthworkers deliver a 'bottom-up' community-based approach, nurses have a more hierarchical 'top-down' biomedical approach. The main concerns for the healthworkers are a lack of respect for their practice and professionalism, and a lack of equality in their relationships with nurses.

At the workshop, the senior manager facilitating the session first summarises the development of the healthworker role. He recalls a campaign by Aboriginal leaders for their people to have different skills and training from nurses 'in order that Aboriginal people would be delivering *Aboriginal* health services'. The manager provides several reasons for the emergence of healthworker programmes: 1) the themes of Aboriginal community control, participation and involvement were then very strong; 2) many Aboriginal communities decided they wanted the stability of locally based healthworkers to counter the transitory nature of nurses; 3) the Nurses Board was unable to facilitate accessible nursing education for Aboriginal people; and 4) nursing courses tended to steer Aboriginal people towards 'mainstream' Australian culture. The Aboriginal leaders' decision that 'We have to train our own mob' prompted the notion of Aboriginal healthworkers and the development of special training programmes.

The manager directed the healthworkers and the nurses to form separate groups to develop descriptions of their respective roles. The terms coined by healthworkers to describe their work include:

client focused / giving people a bit more / catalyst / Jack of all trades, master of none / initial contact / you don't just go and do a job—it's holistic / providing at a grassroots level / day to day / implementing Aboriginal terms of reference / we become a friend—they turn to us / we do it the client's way / we do what they want / service on weekends / a friend / there's no limit / there's no boundary / very broad / no clear role, no clear boundary

Healthworkers describe their role as 'grassroots', responding to the broad day-to-day needs of clients. This is the 'community-based' element of their practice previously articulated by Ruby. However, in relation to other professionals, healthworkers describe their role as being more like a paid servant. According to Sally, 'Nurses do this and

- Jack of all trades, master of none
- providing holistic professional service at a grassroots level
- social welfare, day-to-day basis
- implementing Aboriginal terms of reference
- advocate
- friend/counsellor
- no boundaries (24 hours)
- educator
- no professional role definition of a healthworker

FIGURE 1: The healthworker's role, according to the healthworkers

this, and healthworkers do everything else'. Ruby concurs with her: 'I agree with Sally … our role's not defined … we do what others don't want to do'.

While the healthworkers show some pride in their availability to respond directly to clients, these comments indicate their resentment at being treated barely as assistants by other health professionals. The small group process within the workshop results in a collective formulation of their role (see Figure 1). This description of the healthworker's role, which drew upon their collective practice experience, contrasts markedly with the nurses' description of their role. Their statement is a direct quote from the Nurses Board (see Figure 2).

The healthworkers and nurses approach the definition of their respective roles very differently. While the nurses use a top-down approach, directed and defined bureaucratically, the healthworkers' bottom-up approach is directed and defined by community participation and need. Although previously identified by Ruby in the planning meeting, no one highlights these contrasting approaches within the workshop.

By using the Nurses Board's definition of their role, the nurses not only define their practice but legitimise it in professional terms. Their approach both highlights the lack of a professional governing body for healthworker practice and casts doubt on its legitimacy. While their

---

1 Nursing requires a complex level of behaviours which includes:

- problem solving
- clinical competencies
- co-coordinating abilities
- counsellor
- health teacher
- client advocate
- change agent
- clinical teacher/supervisor
- good communication skills

2 [Nurses Board statement]: A nurse is a person who has completed an approved programme of nurse education and is licensed by a nurse registering authority to practise as a nurse.

FIGURE 2: Nurses Board definition of a registered nurse's role

own activities remain unquestioned, the nurses subsequently scrutinise various healthworker practices. They probe the comprehensiveness of healthworker record-keeping and the legality of other practices, particularly the injecting of clients without supervision.

Whereas the nurses claim their practice domain and support its legitimacy by reference to the Nurses Board, the healthworkers base their claims on the community-based needs of their clients. While no clear demarcation of roles is agreed, professional recognition by other health professionals emerges as a collective concern for the healthworkers.

Structural barriers to recognition and status

The management of the AHS organises a two-day healthworker workshop three months after the combined workshop. The healthworkers use this opportunity to develop a collective definition of a healthworker and to identify their concerns about professional recognition. All eleven qualified healthworkers (other than the team leader of Family Care) attend the workshop.

The focus is on four areas: the definition of a healthworker; the creation of identified healthworker positions within the organisation; the selection processes for healthworkers; and the positioning of healthworkers as first point of contact with clients. Although the healthworkers develop these agenda items prior to the meeting, impetus to shape them as policy proposals comes from a senior manager.

This senior manager, who addresses the healthworkers on the first morning, acknowledges their 'special' ability to work closely with the local Aboriginal people. He identifies them as a 'potentially powerful' group within the AHS and proposes that they need to challenge the mainstream approaches to health care. While he acknowledges that doctors and nurses can offer excellent technical advice within the AHS, he proposes diminishing their roles relative to those of healthworkers. He also observes a need to change the mindset of Aboriginal clients, many of whom prefer services from doctors.

The manager requests proposals on how to promote their role within the AHS and the local Aboriginal community. Noting the agenda item, 'healthworkers as the first point of contact', he requests recommendations concerning the implementation of such a policy. He also encourages the healthworkers to form a small association, to develop a 'healthworker manifesto' for the AHS and to convene a state conference of healthworkers.

Encouraged by this support, the healthworkers share their work experiences over the two days of the workshop. Eventually, following the manager's suggestions, they develop a set of policy proposals and recommendations for implementation within the organisation. Initial discussions focus on qualifications and the definition of a healthworker. The healthworkers express concern that the organisation employs people who lack recognised qualifications, and claim that this results in a negative perception of healthworker practice:

> **Dot**: People are called healthworkers.
> **Rita**: And they're not, they haven't got their certificates.
> **Dot**: [Other health professionals] get the wrong impression from some of these healthworkers that haven't been trained, but

these jobs are going to untrained healthworkers. They're not healthworkers at all.

Ruby: I reckon unless you meet that standard as a healthworker, you shouldn't have that name.

Sally: Same as registered nurses—if you haven't finished your complete registered nurses training.

Ruby: When you do your registration, when you meet the registration board, you have to meet their standards, whether you've done your training at the community level or you've done it at the Healthworker Training College or you've done it at the university. If you can't meet those levels, you're not a healthworker. Let 'em call you something else. Let them call you liaison officer, community worker.

The healthworkers suggest that the labelling of untrained people as Aboriginal healthworkers damages their own professional reputation and standing. Their responses also suggest that they feel slighted by the indifference of the organisation towards their professional qualifications and status. As a result, they propose that within the AHS, only Aboriginal and Torres Strait Islander people with qualifications from an accredited training provider should receive the designation 'Aboriginal health worker'.

The healthworkers indicate that they are deeply offended by the appointment of a woman called Sarina who works in an identified healthworker position without accredited qualifications:

Dot: What happened was [Sarina] said, 'I'm not a healthworker but they employed me as a healthworker, Dot'.

Sally: No, they didn't employ her as a healthworker. Have you seen her duty statement?

Dot: She was officially … she's got no complaints—she said, 'Dot, they chose me for this position'.

Ruby: I don't blame these people because it's the medical team that's doing it, but it was doctors that chose that person, so the doctors are saying we don't value healthworkers, we'll put in who we feel like.

Dot: And Sarina came to me and said they wanted us to train her, and we said we couldn't train Sarina because she's never had any training. How can you train anyone when you are under pressure? You can't. Sarina has no problem—we didn't have a problem.

Rita: But why did she go for it if she wasn't a qualified healthworker?

Ruby: Can I tell you—when we spoke to [the doctor] about it [the doctor] actually said they employed her because she had good management skills.

This example reflects two related concerns: 1) an unqualified person gains the designation 'healthworker'; 2) the selection assumes that it is possible to train a healthworker on the job. According to the healthworkers, such an assumption by management suggests blatant disregard for their hard-earned qualifications. They also suggest that there should be healthworkers on any selection panel assembled for healthworker recruitment, because an experienced and qualified healthworker can assist in both the development of appropriate selection criteria and the assessment of practical skills.

Their final discussion is about healthworkers as the first point of contact with clients. They suggest this would both promote their profile with clients and give them equal status with other healthworkers across the state:

Ruby: This AHS is the only one recently that hasn't employed healthworkers as their main point of contact.

Dot: There's only one healthworker in the clinic, which is myself—one in dental and one in heart health.

Ruby: Every other AHS, when you walk in the door you are seen by a healthworker.

Dot: You see, in the new building we should have three or four screening rooms, and healthworkers there screening the patients before they go to the doctor—that's the need. [The clinic sister] should be there taking blood and doing other stuff as a registered nurse, but the front line should be the healthworker's screening—that's how it should be.

Merle: 'Cause half of the clients don't need to go in and see a doctor, do they.

Sally: How many years have you been the only healthworker there?

Dot: Three.

Sally: Well what's the AHS about if there's only one—you know? I mean, one senior healthworker handling the whole …

Ruby: I think we need to let [the senior manager] know we are not happy with it, 'cause we all just go along and think nothing of it, and he thinks everything is going fine.

Again the healthworkers reveal a perception that management regards healthworkers as marginal to the operations of the AHS.

Towards the end of the two-day workshop, the healthworkers decide to continue to meet as a group. A significant outcome of the workshop is the formation of an ongoing healthworker forum within the AHS, the Indigenous Healthworkers Coalition (IHC).

In summary, this workshop is the first opportunity for all the healthworkers to share their experiences collectively as a professional group. Many experience a lack of respect from nurses and doctors towards their professional experience and training. They identify numerous ways in which organisational structures and procedures marginalise them. By identifying common goals and objectives, the healthworkers achieve some sense of solidarity concerning their professional identity. Their decision to continue to meet as a group under the banner of the IHC further strengthens their solidarity.

The Indigenous Healthworker Coalition

This group met over a period of six months, and initially the focus was on recognition and status. In one of the early IHC meetings, healthworkers indicated that few clients, doctors, nurses or managers have any idea of their training or approach to health service provision. They reiterate their perception that other professionals in the organisation view them negatively:

> **Dot**: I think we've got a real shitty image.
>
> **Rita**: A real jacky ... a lackey jacky, jacky's lackey, a black jacky lackey ... We are the *winyarn*.*
>
> **Dot**: Jack of all trades, but a master of none.
>
> **Ruby**: And AHS doctors and nurses are the worst culprits.
>
> **Rita**: Doctors are the worst.
>
> **Ruby**: Doctors are the worst.

Echoing the combined workshop with nurses described above, the healthworkers perceive that other health professionals treat them almost as servants. They develop a policy that proposes the active promotion of the healthworker role to all AHS staff.

Having a set of written policy proposals and recommendations to enhance professional recognition, the healthworkers discuss strategies for their presentation. The group invites the clinic co-ordinator (a nurse) to attend a meeting. By informing her of their plans and soliciting her ideas, the healthworkers hope to gain her support in AHS management circles for endorsement of their policy recommendations.

Early in the meeting, the chairperson asks the clinic co-ordinator to read the draft policy proposals and provide feedback. Without any consultation, the clinic co-ordinator assumes leadership of the meeting and unilaterally reformulates the proposals. The healthworkers neither challenge her role nor the rewritten proposals.

Afterwards, Ruby expresses her unhappiness at the way the clinic co-ordinator 'dominated' their meeting. With considerable irony, she observes that the same healthworkers have previously claimed professional autonomy:

> We say we want to have our own voice. You should've been there! There was all these *powerful* healthworkers that just agreed to everything [the clinic co-ordinator] said.

---

*A Nyungar expression meaning those who are down and out.

Nevertheless, neither Ruby nor her colleagues had issued a challenge. However, the fact that most healthworkers left before the end of the meeting does indicate some disenchantment with the process.

When the chairperson of the IHC presents the policy recommendations to management, no response is forthcoming. Healthworkers interpret this lack of response as further evidence of their lack of recognition and marginal status.

The IHC also monitors negotiations between the healthworkers union and the AHS concerning a Healthworker Award. The healthworkers perceive that the AHS intends to set their salaries lower than the level proposed for the award. For some, this provides further evidence of their low status within the organisation.

The National Aboriginal and Islander Healthworker Conference is an agenda item of the IHC, and the chairperson announces that the organisers will sponsor her attendance. The IHC organises some fundraising events and, with the support of management, five other healthworkers also attend the conference. This projection of the IHC into a wider forum both before and after the conference shifts the group focus. While initially the focus was on internal organisational matters, with healthworkers outside the AHS expressing interest in joining, the IHC's identity—its purpose, membership and structure—emerges as an issue for the group.

A particular membership problem concerns the Family Care team leader. She is also a healthworker and is a major advocate for healthworkers within the AHS. Initially, she chooses not to be involved in the group so as to enable other voices to be heard, but then she asks to attend the meetings. Though some support her inclusion, most perceive that the more reserved healthworkers participate less readily when she is present. A vote vetoing her participation provokes considerable dissension.

In their early meetings, the healthworkers appear to participate largely as equals. However, the election of their inaugural chairperson changes the participation within the group. Rather than discuss business and formulate direction within the meetings, the chairperson initiates developments independently of the forum. Whereas before the conference, meetings were held fortnightly, after the conference they occur only irregularly.

Shifting morale

Late in my fieldwork, I ask healthworkers individually about their experience of the IHC. Perceptions are very mixed. For some, unanticipated difficulties of coping with the politics of the group result in uneasiness. The lack of response by management has depleted morale. The sharing of information, the openness of meetings and leadership style are among the concerns:

> I didn't see any reason why we couldn't invite a senior manager into the group.

> Is it still going? … I don't know as no one has informed me. We have only had two or three meetings since the conference, and that was three or four months back … You need all the healthworkers, not just handpicked … but they didn't want a middle [management] person. I thought it was a bit much that it happened that way … most probably they needed an older person [as chairperson].

One healthworker reports that the IHC has provided 'Support, encouragement, light at the end of the tunnel, hope', and the value of getting together is appreciated:

> The IHC was helpful with the union thing—it enabled us to access the healthworkers conference—it was good for making sure that jobs were being identified as healthworker specific.

Nevertheless, some healthworkers feel that negative attitudes within the organisation are a major difficulty. These include a view of healthworkers as lower status 'ground' workers and the unwillingness of the organisation to provide time for healthworkers to meet together. One healthworker sums up her experience of the IHC:

I feel like there's things blocking us. Even trying to get strength together, we don't have the support from [the senior manager] or our colleagues. People think healthworkers are the ground workers … people feel [by going to meetings] as though their jobs are on the line … Healthworkers will continue to be less than everyone unless the whole organisation sees us as equal … We feel sad and worthless—I feel that individually … [other people in the organisation] were resentful … Healthworkers have no power here. Your place is there as a healthworker—don't overstep the mark!

In summary, the formation of the IHC provided a unique forum for AHS healthworkers and, in particular, an opportunity to gain professional recognition through their joint efforts. Initially, the forum engendered a strong sense of solidarity and feelings of mutual support. However, political issues arose, including dissension within the group and in relation to some nurses. The associated increase in workplace pressure exposed the healthworkers' lack of professional status and support, tenuous collective identity and fragile professional confidence. They were demoralised by the lack of response by management to their original policy proposals, which sought greater recognition.

INTERACTION, PARTICIPATION AND STATUS

Healthworkers experience difficulties in their professional relationships with both clients and colleagues. The widespread perception among other health professionals that healthworkers are assistants with little status encourages wide-ranging claims on their services. Healthworkers often yield to such claims and seem unwilling to assert their own views either individually or collectively. Furthermore, they find it difficult to engage family members in the care of the elderly, and report widespread exploitative and injurious relationships.

I define injurious relationships with reference to healthworker descriptions of positive working relationships. In a discussion of work ethics, healthworkers identified qualities essential to relationships that they 'enjoyed and felt committed towards' as: respect, trust, understanding, honesty, loyalty and compassion. I therefore define an injurious relationship as one marked by disrespect, mistrust, ignorance, dishonesty, treachery, harm or indifference. In my observation, healthworkers are particularly vulnerable to injurious relationships.

Vulnerability to exploitation and abuse

Home visits expose healthworkers both to the abuse experienced by clients and to being mistreated themselves. For example, clients or family members with complaints sometimes abuse healthworkers verbally on the telephone. In the following case, the healthworkers are aware of the financial abuse of a client by her daughter, and intervention results in serious threats:

> **Patty**: What actually happened is the client, who's homeless, she gives [the Social Security Department] her daughter's address—she's supposed to be staying there. But the daughter gets her pension—the pension goes into her husband's account, who is a white man. So on pension day the client will come to us and say, 'Take me to my daughter, I want to get my pension'. We take her ... the daughter abuses us, tells us, 'You bring her back here again once more, I'll kick all your arses', an' I'll do this, whatever ...
>
> **Ruby**: She actually threatened someone with a knife.
>
> **Patty**: Yes she has—she threatened Christine with a knife.

Healthworkers are not the only staff members vulnerable to abuse by clients and family members. The cleaner reports an instance where, in anticipation of her visit, relatives left their mess for her: 'When I used to go and clean, they'd lay down, and then when I used to get there—they'd leave everything, the dishes, everything'.

A situation arises where glue-sniffing children claim a client's accommodation as a refuge. Upon their eviction, the healthworkers go to clean the house and find human excreta in the rooms, maggots crawling across the floor, filthy mattresses, bedding strewn through the rooms, and hundreds of paint-covered plastic bags and aerosol cans lying about. The Community Development Officer recalls requesting the client to assist:

> He replied, 'You're getting paid for it, you can do it,' and went right on sitting down outside in the sunshine. When I asked him again, he walked inside, picked up one bit of rubbish and walked out again.

I have reported other examples of ill treatment and exploitation of healthworkers, including Rose's acknowledgement that healthworkers run around in circles for clients, and Merle's experience of arriving to transport clients at an appointed time, only to find they are going elsewhere. Clients also request assistance with tasks that healthworkers perceive they can manage for themselves. June reported a request by the social worker to help some clients move house, when she thought they were quite capable of doing it themselves. These examples indicate a level of disrespect, indifference and ignorance towards healthworkers and their practice. I define such relationships between healthworkers and clients as injurious.

When requests for assistance are unreasonable, negotiations founder on the dual role of clients as both service recipients and stakeholders in a community-controlled health service. Some clients translate 'community control' to mean authority over employees, and consequently make ambit claims for assistance. Healthworkers lack clear policy guidelines to negotiate such claims. As a result, Jeanne, the previous field nurse, describes the healthworkers as being 'in turmoil'. Confusion surrounds limits to service provision, and unclear expectations contribute to injurious relationships between healthworkers and clients.

Unreasonable demands may also come from other AHS staff, such as the request from a Welfare worker that June assist clients to move house. As I reported earlier, healthworkers suffer criticism from both Welfare workers and doctors for not cleaning clients' houses or for not ensuring their cleanliness.

Healthworkers are subject to many demands concerning the use of vehicles, and are subject to secondment by the Transport co-ordinator:

> There was stages I was going through when all I did was transport. [The Family Care team leader] would get stuck into me and say, '*Look!*', you know … I'd be doing a job for the [Transport co-ordinator] in the morning or doing something that [the Family Care driver] would normally do and … once they know, they know that you're an easy target or whatever. They'll keep coming back at you and say, 'Oh look, can you do this, can you do that'? I mean, you're own job's lacking, and I got pulled up once or twice about that, because I was neglecting the clients and I was doing more transport than I should be. You've got to put it back on to them.

The holistic nature of healthworker practice, a lack of clear service delivery guidelines, and ignorance about the operations of Family Care within other sections of the AHS expose the healthworkers to inordinate claims on their services. In terms of their criteria for healthy relationships, these claims are injurious inasmuch as they demonstrate disrespect, indifference or ignorance.

A common feature of relationships with other stakeholders in their work is the vulnerability of healthworkers to the agendas or dictates of the other party. Whether in relationship with clients, client family members, co-workers, other health professionals or managers, healthworkers seem to have virtually no basis to assert their own agenda. Both from their own perspective and in the eyes of others, healthworkers have little community, organisational or professional status.

Status and participation in workplace forums

Collective interactions with other health professionals also reveal this lack of status. A particular feature of these interactions is the choice of many healthworkers not to voice their opinions and to remain silent. One possible reason is the arbitrary decision-making style of some managers, which seems to erode healthworker confidence. Paradoxically, some healthworkers in leadership positions also adopt this style.

Best Practice discussions provide some examples of the disincentives to healthworker participation. The sessions aim to clarify policies and procedures and to improve the service delivery of the Family Care section. Staff members share their work experiences, perceptions and practices and, theoretically, all Family Care staff members participate. However, the field nurse and the team leader are not regular participants.

In the first three Best Practice sessions (mostly comprised of healthworkers), staff focus on developing a service delivery protocol. When the team leader finally attends a meeting, rather than participating equally in the discussion with the other healthworkers, she adjudicates their draft proposals from a management standpoint. For example, in the following vignette from the meeting, the team leader, Chronic Care Programme (CCP) co-ordinator and Community Development (CD) officer discuss a proposal to schedule care plan reviews every six months:

> **Researcher** (reading): The care plan will be reviewed by the field nurse, healthworker and client every six months or sooner if required.
>
> **Team leader**: Ummm.
>
> **CD officer**: How about twelve months?
>
> **Team leader**: I was thinking more along the lines of three. Some of our oldies deteriorate fairly quickly.
>
> **CCP co-ordinator**: That's where it says—'sooner if required'. If they have a stroke, if they have a heart attack, if something happens and they need more care.
>
> **Team leader**: OK.
>
> **CCP co-ordinator**: But if nothing's happening, then six months later.
>
> **Team leader**: OK.
>
> **CD officer**: OK.
>
> **Team leader**: That's fine. OK, we'll agree with that one.

Rather than a collaborative stance, the team leader's offer to 'agree' with the draft proposal signals her participation from a management

TABLE 2: Participation in Best Practice meeting

Participant	Proportion of contributions (%)
Team leader	40
Community Development officer	31
Chronic Care Programme co-ordinator	21
Healthworkers (4)	8

Note: The facilitator's input has been excluded.

position. She distances herself from both the participants and authorship of the proposal.

A detailed analysis of the text of this particular meeting reveals the pattern of participation (see Table 2). For the purposes of the analysis, each utterance by a participant in the group is counted as a single contribution. Apart from the Family Care community development worker, all participants are Aboriginal. The proportion of contributions reflects the organisational status of participants. In my perception, the low participation rate of the four healthworkers mirrors their relative lack of status.

A follow-up meeting implements revisions to the proposals. In the absence of both the team leader and the Community Development officer, participant contributions contrast markedly to those in the previous meeting (see Table 3). During this meeting about the same issues all healthworkers participate and demonstrate their concern and interest. This suggests that status is a major factor in low healthworker participation in organisational forums. It indicates that when healthworkers feel free of status differentials, they are able to express their concerns.

Due to the absences of the team leader, the healthworkers realise that the draft Best Practice protocols lack formal recognition. Her absence from the background discussions means that she lacks awareness of the current service delivery issues and therefore of the rationale

TABLE 3: Participation in follow-up meeting

Participant	Proportion of contributions (%)
Healthworkers (4)	56
Chronic Care Programme co-ordinator	37
Cleaner	7

Note: Neither the team leader nor the Community Development officer were present, and the facilitator's input was excluded.

of each protocol. In a joint meeting with the Transport section, the team leader unilaterally overturns a protocol that she has previously endorsed. This action further diminishes healthworker confidence, morale and sense of status.

On another occasion, healthworkers invite the deputy director of the AHS to attend a Best Practice session, where she confronts a catalogue of healthworker concerns about administrative procedures. She inquires whether the meeting was authorised by the Family Care team leader. After assurance that it was, she listens to the healthworkers' concerns. Having rehearsed before the meeting, the healthworkers present their issues with an exceptional degree of confidence. The deputy director indicates that she will respond to their concerns by way of the senior healthworker.

In that meeting, the deputy director adopts a top-down managerial standpoint: she questions the authorisation for the meeting and offers to respond through line management. During discussions between healthworkers after the meeting, Josie suggests that in the presence of the deputy director, the 'atmosphere' of the meeting had changed. Merle observes that the deputy director gave the impression she was reluctant to talk with the staff. Ruby perceives that she made excuses for the administration team. I observe that the healthworkers seem uncomfortable with the managerial style of the deputy director. Again, they appear to have difficulty expressing opinions and concerns in organisational forums in the presence of managers. Despite their experience and knowledge, healthworkers display little confidence in their own status, in management's regard for their proposals and in the value of their participation.

The association between status and participation is thus clearly evident at meetings of the IHC. Initially, each of the healthworkers has a share in the ownership of the group and participation is strong. They choose someone to chair their meetings, and that chairperson, like some other managers, displays an arbitrary style of leadership. She frequently makes decisions without consulting her fellow healthworkers who, in her presence, seem lacking in confidence and unwilling to challenge. This provides yet another example of the hesitancy of the healthworkers, even collectively, to assert their opinions in the face of anyone with management or leadership status. It also indicates their lack of morale as a professional group.

A TENUOUS PROFESSIONAL IDENTITY

Family Care healthworkers themselves perceive the 'Family Care healthworker' as a unique professional with a distinct practice—a practice based in the community, engaged with the lives of clients and derived from both specific training and their own Aboriginality. According to them, their practice embraces an alternative frame of reference to that of doctors and nurses: community need determines both the orientation and legitimacy of their practice. In contrast, they perceive that the biomedical model determines the practice of other health professionals, whose legitimacy is derived from professional boards. On the basis of these distinctions, healthworkers claim a unique professional status and identity.

Nevertheless, seldom are their claims to professional status acknowledged by their colleagues. Prime examples are the continuing attempts by other professionals and managers to co-opt them. According to healthworkers, doctors give scant recognition to social factors, such as client mobility, mistrust and disruption, as major contributors to lack of adherence to treatment schedules. Likewise, they perceive that nurses treat them as if they are ignorant. Rarely are healthworkers invited to be genuine participants in AHS policy and programme planning, despite their close links to the community. Lack of recognition saps their morale.

Despite statements about the key role of Aboriginal healthworkers in the field of Aboriginal health, these healthworkers find that their lack of professional status within their organisation gives them the scope to 'change nothing'. Not only do other health professionals ultimately determine their contribution, but in practical terms the management is unable to support them. Lacking support to develop solidarity, the healthworkers become subject to even greater pressures. As a result of these experiences, this group of healthworkers expresses serious disillusionment about their professional role, their value to their organisation and their capacity to contribute to the field of Aboriginal health in general. In the next chapter, I outline their central dilemmas, examine how their experiences compare with those of Aboriginal healthworkers generally, and offer some proposals for a way forward.

CHAPTER — 5

Genesis of a Healing Practice?

The accounts in previous chapters reveal disparate perceptions about healthworker practice and some key dilemmas—not only for healthworkers, but also for other health professionals and, potentially, for policy-makers. I will now examine four key issues emergent from these accounts, compare them with other observations and analysis of healthworker practice, and discuss the implications for future policy. The literature indicates that the experiences of outreach healthworkers outlined here would resonate with clinic-based Indigenous healthworkers and those in other settings.

I suggest that the unique client-centred holistic approach of the healthworkers in this study offers a way forward. Institutional acknowledgement and endorsement of this approach would strengthen the effectiveness of healthworkers.

KEY HEALTHWORKER EXPERIENCES

Lack of clarity and continuing contestation amongst health professionals and educators about the practice of Aboriginal healthworkers motivated this ethnographic study of their lived reality and day-to-day practice. The central question is, how do healthworkers engaged at the frontline of Aboriginal health service delivery understand the suffering they encounter and their role in addressing it?

Four key facets of Family Care healthworker experience are identi-fied within this study: 1) the contextual complexity of day-to-day engagement with both clinical and social problems, 2) a unique and distinctive client-centred holistic practice, 3) their marginal profess-ional status, and 4) the effect of the barely recognised conjunction of these factors in creating strain and pressure and eroding morale.

The contextual complexities

Within Aboriginal households, healthworkers attempt daily to engage and assist clients to manage serious chronic diseases—diabetes, respira-tory disease, heart disease, arthritis and renal disease—and associated conditions. Almost inevitably, the healthworkers despair at the frequency with which clients seem unable to maintain the necessary regimens of care. Consistently, they encounter clients mismanaging their health conditions and maintaining potentially dangerous blood pressure and blood sugar levels. Many of their clients live at high risk of stroke, heart attack, blindness, disability and death.

Significant obstacles confront the healthworkers' attempts to support clients in their management of chronic illnesses. Environmen-tal, social and cultural factors, often related to marginalisation and poverty, undermine the health of clients and their capacity to manage illness. Even small successes, such as convincing clients to adopt simple systems of medication scheduling, are dwarfed by endemic social disruption—cash and food shortages, inadequate housing, high unem-ployment, low education levels, widespread alcohol and substance abuse, social security issues, custodial issues, domestic violence and welfare dependency.

As many clients ignore their own clinical health problems in their efforts to reconcile disruptions to their living situation, healthworkers inevitably become embroiled in the struggle. For instance, overcrowded and chaotic households undermine attempts by sick and disabled clients to control their diabetes. Compromised by tough realities, the healthworkers despair at their fruitless attempts to encourage clients to manage their health, and some accord their efforts the status of 'bandaid' treatments.

Disparate client priorities are just one reason for a lukewarm response to healthworker efforts. According to the healthworkers, historical experiences of racism and exclusion are instrumental to the clients' general lack of education and the widespread mistrust of health professionals. Half-hearted client responses discourage healthworker attempts to engage them in prevention and education programmes. The effort required to overcome the scars of history—fear, mistrust and dependency—is in itself a substantial assignment.

Client dependency presents another significant challenge to the skills and morale of the healthworkers. In the midst of widespread social disruption, the healthworkers find themselves negotiating wide-ranging claims on their services. Caught in a dilemma between providing ines-sential services in order to strengthen client trust and enabling clients to 'stand on their own two feet', healthworkers grapple with the contemporary outcomes of a legacy of imposed welfare dependency. Where dependency extends to exploitation and abuse within families, health-workers confront an even greater struggle. Intervention in an abuse case is a risky and complex entanglement for healthworkers, due to insufficient organisational support and their vulnerability, as community members, to 'payback'.

The unique situation of healthworkers, with their dual status as community members and health service providers, and their painful familiarity with the contextual complexities facing clients, prompted the development of a distinct professional practice.

A unique practice

The healthworkers' client-centred holistic practice emerges as a specific, pragmatic response to factors that undermine the health of their clients. The practitioners embody particular values, ways of relating, intervention priorities and ways of working. In addition to a limited clinical component, their practice encompasses environmental, social, psychosocial and cultural aspects of wellbeing—health determinants which healthworkers perceive are often ignored. In addition, unlike non-Aboriginal professional colleagues, healthworkers relate to clients using Aboriginal social and cultural *mores* and an informal, grassroots style.

While the healthworkers explicitly distinguish respect, trust, understanding, honesty and loyalty as important values within their professional relationships, also implicit within their practice are compassion, openness and flexibility. They engage an informal style of relationship in order to diminish client mistrust, so that health messages can 'get through' to clients. In a context of endemic social disruption and uncertainty, such relationships with professionals seemed remarkable to some clients, such as one who confessed, 'I feel guilty, they look after me so well'.

A central component of the healthworkers' practice is that of a middleman, whereby they facilitate client relationships with other health service providers. However, the broad scope of their practice amongst high levels of need often means that they are besieged by multiple, disparate and immediate client demands. Other health professionals also recognise the middleman role, and engage the healthworkers, perceiving that they are Jacks of all trades. Their status as assistants further complicates their task and confuses healthworker priorities.

Despite the difficulties inherent in their unique approach, their distinct practice provides the foundation for healthworker claims for a professional identity distinct from the largely clinical domain of doctors and nurses. As unique community-based practitioners, the healthworkers perceive that they offer a significant and valuable perspective to the field of Aboriginal health in general and, in particular, to health policy and planning processes.

Marginal professional status

Despite their unique practice and potential contribution to planning, healthworkers receive scant professional recognition in their day-to-day work. While the complexities of their practice in the community are evident to other outreach staff, few doctors or nurses acknowledge it and most maintain a narrow, clinical view of healthworker practice. Doctors generally perceive healthworkers as medical extension workers engaged in providing simple clinical monitoring, health education services and health surveillance. They maintain that healthworkers should supply them with relevant, social, cultural and environmental information to supplement clinical assessment. Not only do doctors and nurses view healthworkers primarily as adjuncts to clinical practice but also, on the basis of clinical criteria, they judge them as somewhat incompetent.

The healthworkers in this study experience considerable frustration with the narrow clinical conceptualisation of their practice. They argue that by restricting their practice to clinical health, scant credence is granted to the substantial environmental, social and cultural factors that constitute major health risks for their clients. Furthermore, they find that health professionals holding a solely clinical view of their practice often lack awareness of the nature and depth of healthworker/client relationships, and sometimes undermine these relationships unknowingly or judge them as 'unprofessional'. Consequently, significant tension often exists between the healthworkers and the doctors and nurses. With few exceptions, both doctors and nurses perceive little that is special about healthworker practice, and accord healthworkers no significant status in the professional health hierarchy.

Healthworkers claim that they are granted negligible professional recognition, not only from other professionals but also from their employing organisation. While some individual managers extol healthworker practice and status, contrary actions by management as a whole signal the opposite. The healthworkers suggest that the organisation has no criteria to govern the designation 'healthworker', and that managers disregard their qualifications, fail to orient other staff to their role, exclude them from policy and programme planning and ignore their policy proposals. They complain that in organisational terms, they are 'lackeys'. Perceiving themselves as marginal, both professionally and organisationally, many therefore avoid voicing their concerns in broader organisational forums.

The lack of professional recognition from colleagues carries over into relationships with clients. Just as colleagues make unregulated demands on healthworkers as low-status workers, clients too make spurious claims. By responding, the healthworkers risk fostering client dependency; by not responding, they may jeopardise their relationship with the client. Faced with these dilemmas amidst heavy client demand, these healthworkers developed a definitive set of service guidelines.

Assaults on morale

Healthworkers are at the juncture of a complex set of demands and expectations from both clients and other health professionals. At almost every turn, they face a plethora of personal and professional challenges. Not surprisingly, these varied and persistent challenges adversely affect morale.

In separate community, organisational and professional contexts, the healthworkers encounter disparate ideas about their work. Managers, doctors, nurses, welfare workers, transport drivers and clients all espouse particular ideas of what healthworkers should do—ideas based mostly on their own priorities. The healthworkers' conceptions of their work also vary, depending on the particular emphasis of their training. However, they lack organisational endorsement of their own draft service guidelines, and the diverse claims on their time pull the healthworkers in many directions.

The grave health status of their community confronts healthworkers daily. Their engagement with serious chronic illnesses and endless environmental, social and cultural problems is continuous and unrelenting—and is further ruptured and fragmented by client fear, mistrust, conflicting priorities, exploitation, abuse and dependency. Such day-to-day realities place a burden on healthworker morale, and awareness that their genesis is in larger social forces producing poverty, exclusion and racism further taxes their commitment.

Frequent challenges to the healthworkers' standing as health professionals from colleagues, clients and management deplete zeal further. Evaluation of their practice by clinical criteria, misinterpretation and depreciation of their professional judgement, marginalisation by organisational structures and processes, and perception of them as potential assistants are common experiences which impel healthworkers to question their dedication.

Astonishingly, the healthworkers within this study nevertheless devoted considerable time to working together as a group and formulating practice guidelines to enable them to work effectively, safely and with the necessary organisational support. In the face of extraordinary obstacles, they also developed and articulated a unique style of practice, which they perceived would make a difference to the lives of their clients. And all the while, they maintained their services.

The focus of this study on just fourteen healthworkers may bring into question the validity of the findings. Do the experiences and perspectives presented here represent those of only a minority of healthworkers, or do they indicate broad systemic issues? An exploration of the literature suggests that confusion and conflict about the role of Aboriginal healthworkers has been present from the beginning. Previous reports indicate negligible consideration of healthworker practice within the social and cultural context of Aboriginal ill health, and a clear gap between workforce policy and actual practice is evident. Consistently, reports indicate that like Family Care healthworkers, many other Aboriginal healthworkers encounter similar difficulties.

ABORIGINAL HEALTHWORKERS ELSEWHERE

Healthworker practice has long been the subject of debate and even controversy. The practice of some healthworkers is broad, while that of others has very limited scope. Policy often bears negligible resemblance to actual service delivery. Examination of the literature indicates that few planners or researchers consider healthworker practice in terms of the complex environmental, social and cultural factors impinging on the health of clients. While some literature highlights healthworker concerns about low status, less attention is directed to the resultant low morale and large numbers of resignations.

Divergent conceptions of practice

Since the beginning, divergent conceptions of healthworker practice have produced enduring confusion and debate. Within the AHS, views of clinical health professionals diverge from those of healthworkers. What I have described as a client-centred holistic practice places healthworkers at odds with most doctors and nurses, who advocate a narrow clinical approach. Congruent with the literature presented below, AHS doctors, nurses and even general staff perceive healthworkers as auxiliaries rather than as practitioners in their own right.

As indicated in Chapter 1, the literature indicates that other health personnel frequently perceive healthworker practice as a way to achieve their own ends. Government health planners have constructed health-worker roles in line with the politics of Aboriginal self-management; nurses with clinical responsibilities have moulded healthworker practice with a clinical orientation; advocates of primary health care have described healthworker practice in broad terms. Over the years, in many diverse situations, healthworkers have thus encountered conflicting understandings and expectations of their role.[1]

The widespread understanding of healthworkers as 'cultural brokers' has also been contested. Soong, a doctor in the early Northern Territory healthworker programme, promoted this specific linking role. He envisaged four activities of healthworkers as cultural brokers: 'acting as the main source of information for clients; acting as the main source of information about community and clients for nurses; changing the expectations and practices of the client; and, changing expectations and behaviours of the nurses'.[2] Subsequently, Tregenza and Abbott, and Willis, have suggested that 'cultural broking' primarily serves the pur-poses and interests of clinical professionals, rather than being a two-way relationship that also serves the client's interest.[3]

The healthworkers within this study also identify 'linking' or brok-ering as a crucial and central component of their practice. In marked contrast to the conception of Soong, their middleman role primarily services the client's interest. They describe their practice as client-centred. In contrast, AHS doctors and nurses retain Soong's idea of healthworkers as brokers in service to clinical priorities. The healthwork-ers base their middleman role on an Aboriginal style of relationship—a practice previously advocated by Anderson.[4]

During the 1990s conceptualisations of healthworker practice at higher policy levels broadened, subsequent to Anderson's groundbreak-ing book, *Koorie Health in Koorie Hands* (1988) and the publication of the first National Aboriginal Health Strategy.[5] Both espoused an Aboriginal 'whole of life' view of health. However, at the point of service delivery, the literature reveals that the professional orientation of colleagues and the demands of clients largely determine healthworker practice. Within remote community clinics, in the face of clinical demands and alongside clinical practitioners, healthworker practice has been mostly clinical.[6]

In contrast, the urban situation reported in this study shows that in the face of wide-ranging social demands and under the leadership of a relatively highly trained healthworker, healthworker practice can be more holistic. While Family Care healthworker practice is also subject to many interpretations, its client-centred holistic approach, directed towards broader contextual factors, echoes the aspiration of many healthworkers in a variety of contexts.[7]

Masking the complexities?

While numerous government reports have revealed both the widespread poverty and the poor health status of Aboriginal people,[8] the impact of related environmental, social and cultural factors on healthworker practice has received little serious consideration. Only in the last decade have questions arisen about the complexity and range of the health-worker task.

While Josif and Elderton, and Franks and Curr, have reported healthworkers feeling overwhelmed by both the seriousness of clinical demands and the magnitude of the task,[9] concerns have been raised more recently, for the most part by Aboriginal health professionals.[10] Flick has suggested that healthworkers are engaged on the frontline of a seemingly endless battle:

> More of our people die of preventable diseases each year than Australian troops killed in the whole of the Vietnam War, and these numbers are increasing year by year. And, as all of us know, it is the Aboriginal health workers who are in the frontline of this struggle. It is the Aboriginal Health Workers who face, day in, day out the continuing tragedy of our ill health.[11]

Likewise, some healthworkers in this study report feeling 'numb' in the face of frequent client deaths, and disheartened in the face of a 'never-ending story' of ill health.

While the magnitude of clinical morbidity and, in particular, serious chronic disease creates significant demands, healthworkers in a wide range of contexts have suggested that broader factors related to marginalisation and poverty also require attention.[12] However, where healthworkers are situated in clinics as clinical assistants, many clients identify healthworkers solely with clinical practice.[13] A particular emphasis on clinical ailments, amidst widespread client mistrust and lack of confidence, suggests that broader problems affecting an individual's health are unlikely to be raised.

In remote communities, the likelihood of a clinical orientation that deflects attention from broader environmental, social and cultural health factors integral to client wellbeing may be particularly strong. As remote area healthworkers have few resources at hand to address broader health factors they may, for instance, be less able to represent or stand alongside clients in face-to-face encounters with local welfare and housing agencies.

In contrast, within the urban context, healthworkers engage directly with many of the broader issues of deprivation and marginalisation, and many urban clients give these issues priority. Moreover, in the urban context, some healthworkers engage the underlying factors associated with these broader issues, such as fear, mistrust, dependency, exploitation and abuse.

Related to this mistrust and fear, and adding further complexity to the healthworker task, are the dispirited responses of clients. Healthworkers encounter client mistrust towards health professionals in a range of contexts.[14] Many Family Care clients mistrust doctors and are unwilling to attend either clinic consultations or hospital. Josif and Elderton also report mistrust and a lack of responsiveness among clients in the Northern Territory. According to healthworkers in their study, clients were unwilling to seek care and were not interested in health education:

[The job is] getting people to see the doctor …

Doctor can be here all day and people won't come and visit—wait till doctor gone and then they'll come, because frightened of doctor—they don't want to see white people …

You're trying to educate people in health matters and people aren't interested.[15]

Widespread mistrust of healthworkers was also reported at the 1997 National Aboriginal and Torres Strait Islander Healthworker Conference:

Many delegates complained that they are forced to deal with mistrust on a daily basis. Communities required a great deal of groundwork to build up levels of trust and begin to accept the various types of service and treatments offered by Western models of health care.[16]

Client 'resistance' has been documented by other observers.[17] And accounts from the Northern Territory report many healthworkers with insufficient community status to discharge their duties. Soong reported healthworkers using the endorsement of the nurse to influence clients by, for example, saying 'Sister wants you'.[18]

Where healthworkers lack status and community support, they are reluctant to implement health education and environmental programmes.[19] McMasters, a healthworker himself, has observed that it is often difficult to provide advice and health information to clients when it is interpreted as interference, telling people what to do, or personal criticism.[20] The healthworkers within this study also have difficulty engaging clients in such programmes, particularly those directed towards lifestyle changes.

While the complexities of the healthworker task in the face of client mistrust and lack of responsiveness have received some attention in the literature, this is not the case for the client dependency identified by healthworkers within this study. Although kinship obligations are widely acknowledged to influence healthworker service delivery,[21] few studies reveal the subtleties of healthworker/client interaction. Notably absent in the healthworker literature is the difficult practice of discriminating and negotiating essential need, and of encouraging clients to 'take control' of their own health within a context of systemic welfare dependency.

Another complex challenge largely unacknowledged in the literature is the exploitation and abuse of clients. The healthworkers in this study have serious concerns about the detrimental effects of childcare on elderly clients with serious chronic illnesses, a problem also reported by Tregenza and Abbott.[22] When confronting serious cases of financial, physical, emotional and sexual abuse, healthworkers often encounter a code of silence, become acutely conscious of their community identity, and fear 'payback' should they expose a perpetrator. While the literature documents fears of blaming and revenge in the face of unsuccessful treatments, reports of abuse and the associated fears are rare (an exception is Windsor).[23]

Consequently, a crucial cultural issue with the potential to complicate the healthworkers' task further is their own identity as members of the community. This exposes the healthworker to significantly different pressures from those faced by an outside health professional. Crucially, it exposes them to family pressures,[24] as well as to similar health risks and social problems as their clients. According to Tregenza and Abbott, many healthworkers 'are themselves sick or have relatives who are sick and for whom they must care',[25] a situation which is seldom understood by non-Aboriginal staff. Tsey indicates that the low level of education and literacy among Northern Territory healthworkers reflects a situation common within their own communities.[26]

In summary, while Family Care healthworkers encounter many cases of serious chronic illnesses and a chaotic mix of social and cultural problems related to social exclusion and poverty, seldom are these contextual complexities explicitly acknowledged in reports concerning healthworkers. Although reports have revealed client mistrust, lack of responsiveness and resistance, and healthworkers' lack of community status and exposure to similar health risks as their clients, two key experiences of Family Care healthworkers are largely missing. These are 1) in the context of systemic welfare dependency, the need to identify genuine need and to encourage clients to take control of their own health; and 2) fears of revenge and payback in their encounters with exploitation and abuse within client families.

Professional confusion and exclusion

Foremost among the considerable difficulties faced by Family Care healthworkers in relating to the professional context of their practice is a lack of professional recognition and status.

At the level of service delivery, it is evident that most healthworkers have minimal status. Since programmes first began, it appears that doctors and nurses have conceptualised and evaluated healthworker practice primarily in clinical terms. Further, because most nurses are subordinate to doctors, they place healthworkers even lower in the health hierarchy. Accounts in the literature parallel a key finding in this study: that decision-making processes exclude healthworkers.

Within the literature, however, the centrality of healthworkers to the delivery of Aboriginal health services has been consistently promoted at higher policy levels. Soong advocated the potential of healthworker practice in the Northern Territory,[27] and his fellow doctors posited healthworkers as being critical to the delivery of services. For example, Hargrave described healthworkers as the 'linchpin' of service delivery.[28] Similarly, Devanesen, and Fleming and Devanesen promoted the Northern Territory healthworker programme as the 'key' to Aboriginal self-determination and self-management in health.[29] In another context, Anderson stressed healthworkers as being a vital link between professional staff and the local Aboriginal community.[30] The National Aboriginal Health Strategy Working Party identified the Aboriginal healthworker programme as 'one of the most important factors in efforts to improve Aboriginal health status'.[31]

During the 1990s the importance of the 'key' healthworker role was advocated consistently at higher policy levels,[32] to the point of being 'crucial'[33] and 'pivotal',[34] and the emphasis was on professional registration, career structures, accredited training and the portability of qualifications. Underlying these initiatives is an assumption that healthworker practice is a distinct body of work. As a consequence, healthworkers were removed from nursing line-management in both the Northern Territory and Western Australia.[35] Nevertheless, at the level of service delivery, nurses, clients and healthworkers themselves experienced confusion about their status and practice.[36]

A striking feature within the literature is the continued conflict and confusion about healthworker practice since its inception. Soong provides an early account of miscommunication, misinterpretation of policy, and conflicts between health professionals developing the Northern Territory healthworker programme.[37] These conflicts concerned training methods, curriculum, recruitment and practice. In Western Australia, Hart observed confusion among health professionals.[38] And Armstrong et al. suggested that professionals in the Aboriginal Affairs bureaucracy, government and non-government health agencies all had differing perceptions of healthworker practice.[39]

Early ideas about a broad role for healthworkers in the Northern Territory healthworker programme, as outlined in Chapter 1, were at odds with the predominantly clinical focus of their practice—alongside nurses acting both as their supervisors and mentors. Soong, Dixon et al. and Willis, all noted that most nurses qualified neither as practitioners nor as advisers about a comprehensive primary health care approach.[40] Soong observed that being dependent on nurses for clinical knowledge and skills meant that healthworkers 'appeared to be disadvantaged in power terms', and a similar situation was reported in Western Australia.[41] Nevertheless, the literature records that claims for the professional equivalence of healthworkers have been advocated since the early 1980s.[42]

In parallel with the experience of Family Care healthworkers, the literature indicates that nurses generally accord healthworkers lower professional status. Kirkby reported that 'In most instances the health worker assists the nurse, follows her/his lead, obeys his/her instructions and works to her/his plan'.[43] Similarly to reports concerning primary health workers in the international context, Australian nurses have generally treated Aboriginal healthworkers as their clinical assistants, evaluated them using clinical criteria and found them wanting.[44] Jackson observed that nurses co-opt healthworkers into the lower levels of the rigid hierarchy of status within nursing, a process that most nurses experience themselves.[45] Likewise, Tregenza and Abbott, and Windsor, reported that healthworkers feel they are placed at the bottom of the power pyramid, below nurses and doctors.[46]

In parallel with the nurses' perceptions of healthworkers within this study, Tregenza and Abbott reported that nurses feel that employers overstate the healthworker role and that this rhetoric contradicts the reality.[47] Bradley reported unfulfilled expectations and confusion about healthworkers' practice in her remote nursing experience.[48]

In brief, the evidence from this study about the central and problematic relationship between healthworkers and nurses receives abundant support from the literature. Essentially, in a wider context of confusion amongst clinical professionals about healthworker practice, nurses frequently become the supervisors or mentors of clinical health-worker practice. The limited clinical competence of healthworkers often means that nurses treat them as subordinates rather than equals. Healthworkers holding a broader view of health have found themselves out of step, out of place and lacking professional status. As a result, their potential contribution has rarely been understood or acknowledged. Within this study, attempts by healthworkers to institute a set of practice guidelines to overcome lack of acknowledgement of their client-centred holistic approach remain ignored and unsupported by their own organisation.

Despite the rhetoric at higher policy levels, there is consistent evidence since healthworker programmes began of the marginal community and professional status of healthworkers. Nathan and Japanangka noted that healthworkers lacked the status of either doctors or traditional healers.[49] Widespread and ongoing reports of inadequate in-service training and professional development opportunities for healthworkers also indicated marginal status.[50]

Josif and Elderton have reported that healthworkers within the Northern Territory health department were 'largely ignored in the policy formulation and implementation process'.[51] Franks and Curr suggested that a major reason for dissatisfaction among healthworkers was their lack of equivalent status with other health professionals, a perception also reported by Dollard et al.[52] Flick described the incongruous position of healthworkers 'whose local cultural knowledge has been accumulated over decades of living and working with their people being completely ignored when it comes to health planning carried out by the experts'.[53] Likewise, healthworkers in Central Australia felt they could not effectively link the community and the health service without being included in policy and programme development.[54] Hecker also reported the exclusion of healthworkers from planning and decision-making in a participatory study with healthworkers in northern South Australia.[55]

Scrimgeour observed that healthworkers have negligible organisational status even within non-government Aboriginal health services.[56] He reported that the spokespeople on Aboriginal health issues are generally Aboriginal managers rather than healthworkers, and noted the resistance of the peak organisation for Aboriginal Health Services, the National Aboriginal Controlled Community Health Organisation, towards the formation of a national healthworker organisation.

In essence, congruent with the experience of the healthworkers in this study, the literature indicates that in most contexts healthworkers have lacked professional recognition, organisational status and influence in the Aboriginal health arena. It is apparent that widespread confusion is generated by the promotion at higher policy levels of healthworker practice as being pivotal, while contrary perceptions prevail at the level of service delivery. Similarly, as in the literature, most nurses within this study report confusion about healthworkers, evaluate healthworker practice in clinical terms and place them low on the professional health hierarchy.

The low status of healthworkers in professional terms is paralleled in organisational terms. As in this study, healthworkers in a variety of contexts have understood that at the policy level their role is seen as both broad in scope and pivotal in importance. However, most experience lower organisational status than other health professionals, and exclusion from policy and programme planning. In this respect, the situation of the Family Care healthworkers is a microcosm of healthworker experiences generally.

High resignation rates, low morale

The morale of healthworkers is sorely tested by their uncertain professional status amidst daily engagement with the suffering of their own people and families.

The literature has indicated that in a wide range of contexts, pressures from a variety of sources undermine healthworker morale. These pressures include the unrelenting demand for clinical services due to endemic serious chronic illnesses, client resistance to prevention programmes, conflict between community and professional expectations, and the lack of recognition, respect and status. Similar pressures faced by healthworkers within this study provoked them to question their commitment to their work. Such concerns have consistently resulted in high resignation rates from healthworker programmes generally.

High resignation rates have been reported in the literature for at least twenty years. Hart reported that in the Health Department of Western Australia, 46 per cent of healthworkers resigned in their first year of service and 22 per cent in their second year. The numbers declined from 97 healthworkers in 1986 to 79 Full Time Equivalents in 1996.[57] Kirkby reported that while she was unable to determine the drop-out rate in the Kimberley region, perceptions of workers in the field indicated that the figure was high.[58]

Northern Territory statistics describe similar trends. In 1979, 300 healthworkers were employed by Northern Territory Health.[59] A 1991 report showed that only 70 per cent of funded Aboriginal healthworker positions were filled (i.e. 216 positions or 165.15 Full Time Equivalents),[60] and suggested that a 30 per cent shortfall of healthworkers was hampering primary health care services in rural communities. While many of the difficulties faced by healthworkers had already been documented,[61] the Northern Territory Health Department commissioned two reports on their recruitment and retention.[62] Subsequently, Tregenza and Abbot confirmed many earlier findings.[63]

Hart suggested that a lack of clarity among doctors, nurses and healthworkers about the focus of the healthworker role was probably the most important factor in healthworker resignations.[64] Almost fifteen years later Tregenza and Abbott, and Hecker, reported similar findings—in particular, the frustration of healthworkers at their exclusion from a key role in service delivery outside the clinic.[65]

Tregenza and Abbott, along with Dixon et al., have indicated that healthworkers perceive that medical and nursing staff lack commitment towards the healthworker programme.[66] Josif and Elderton reporting on the Northern Territory, and Kirkby reporting on northern Western Australia, noted that healthworkers lack organisational support, supervision and training.[67] Tregenza and Abbott echoed Josif and Elderton's assertion that tension exists between healthworkers and nurses, and that healthworkers lack status, an issue also reported by Franks and Curr, and Hecker.[68] Along with Kirkby,[69] all these reports indicated frustration among healthworkers who are confined to clinical duties in communities where, alongside the high clinical demand, environmental, social and cultural issues are major determinants of health status.

Reports by Dixon, Kelly and Kirke, and Franks and Curr indicated healthworker frustration at the lack of cultural awareness of non-Aboriginal staff, particularly concerning the community obligations of healthworkers.[70] Hart, Dixon et al., Josif and Elderton, Franks and Curr, and Tregenza and Abbott, all indicated that healthworkers face considerable stress due to cultural obligations, the magnitude of community demands and their relatively greater exposure to these compared to non-Aboriginal staff.[71] Josif and Elderton particularly stressed the pressure felt by healthworkers due to the fear of payback for unsuccessful treatments.[72]

These reports of the numerous factors affecting healthworker morale echo the findings within this study. At the service delivery level, healthworkers engage highly complex clinical, environmental, social and cultural determinants of health. Furthermore, membership of the community often places additional complications on healthworker practice. While at the policy level, healthworkers are projected as pivotal, in the workplace they have minimal status and are marginalised from policy planning. Consequently, many healthworkers become demoralised and choose to resign.

IMPLICATIONS AND RECOMMENDATIONS

I suggest that amidst historical misunderstandings, confused expectations and the contextual complexities associated with Aboriginal clients, two distinct models of practice have emerged: the clinical assistant, or the broader practitioner focused predominantly on prevention. The client-centred holistic practice described within this study in many ways resembles the latter model, and is a conception that has endured since healthworker programmes first began. Along with the participants of this study, I suggest that a client-centred holistic practice, adequately integrated and supported, can strengthen Aboriginal health services. Potentially it provides accessible, acceptable and culturally appropriate services for clients, responds to persistent calls for an emphasis on primary prevention and provides the foundation for a distinct Indigenous professional health practice.

Reconciling disparate conceptions

Strikingly apparent historically, and conspicuous within this study is the continuing poor health status of Aboriginal people. Working at the grassroots level in the homes of their clients, this is patently manifest to Aboriginal healthworkers. They continually engage clients who are at the mercy of and entangled with a synergistic mix of damaging clinical, social, environmental and cultural factors. These factors also work to limit access to mainstream health services, thus compounding the problems.

In historical terms, enhancement of access to health services has been the central rationale for the employment of Aboriginal healthworkers. According to the National Aboriginal Health Strategy, healthworkers 'bridge the cultural chasm enabling two-way communication between clients and the mainstream health system'.[73] The employment of healthworkers is a response to similar recommendations within the Alma Ata Declaration on Primary Health Care: to make health services more accessible, acceptable and culturally appropriate.[74]

Following earlier and influential World Health Organization definitions, the Alma Ata Declaration significantly influenced the scope of healthworker practice by defining health broadly, as 'a state of complete physical, mental and social well being, and not merely the absence of disease or infirmity'.[75] Likewise, the original National Aboriginal Health Strategy and the 2003 National Strategic Framework for Aboriginal and Torres Strait Islander Health promote a holistic conception of Aboriginal health: 'Not just the physical well-being of the individual but the social, emotional, and cultural wellbeing of the whole community … a "whole of life" view'.[76] A broad health practice was advocated for primary health workers within the international health context.[77] Echoing the Alma Ata Declaration, definitions of Aboriginal health-worker practice embraced not only clinical issues, but also broader social health determinants.[78]

Nevertheless, some experts queried the recommendations of Alma Ata, particularly advocates of selective primary health care, who promoted the implementation of vertical programmes—that is, those that addressed particular diseases. They challenged the advocates of comprehensive primary health care programmes and their broad, integrated, multi-sectorial approach.[79] Similarly, the literature records disparate views about the conception and scope of the UNICEF and World Health Organization vision of primary health worker practice,[80] and of Aboriginal healthworkers in the Australian context.[81]

As suggested above, two distinct models of healthworker practice have emerged. One model frames a healthworker primarily as a clinical extension worker: someone who visits clients in the community, dresses wounds, monitors vital signs and medication use, provides health information, provides referrals and undertakes surveillance of social and environmental health determinants.

The other model describes healthworkers as broad or holistic practitioners who, in addition to simple clinical tasks, initiate preventive action on environmental, social and cultural health determinants. Generally, the holistic approach includes a client-centred case focus on basic clinical care, support, advocacy and health education. It sometimes also includes a community focus, initiating broader action on health education, action and development.

The clinical conceptualisation of Aboriginal healthworker practice is dominant in many contexts and is usually the perspective of doctors and nurses. Within remote communities, where rates of clinical morbidity are often extremely high, many healthworkers report that their narrow clinical role largely confines them to duties as a nurse's assistant in the clinic. Likewise, within clinics at larger population centres, their practice is reportedly mainly clinical and confined to assisting other health professionals.

While most AHS doctors acknowledge that Aboriginal healthworkers relate readily to their own people, the clinical view is that healthworkers provide a service that could equally be received by a non-Aboriginal person. Whether delivered in the community or the clinic, this narrow clinical practice meets the criteria for an accessible, acceptable and culturally appropriate practice almost solely through the identity of the Indigenous practitioner. This view of what constitutes an appropriate service for Aboriginal people is rendered somewhat superficial by the results of this study.

This study has shown that the provision of appropriate and effective health services for Aboriginal people is not merely a technical exercise, a matter of enacting clinical routines, relaying pre-packaged health messages and transporting prescription pharmaceuticals. Health care in this context means establishing a trusting relationship with the client, assuaging their fears of the health system and bolstering their confidence so as to enable them to take control of their own health. In addition, health care includes reducing the pressure of social disruptions in clients' lives so that they have the space to attend to their own personal health needs. Moreover, health care involves strengthening family support. The practitioners in this study attempted to deliver a client-centred holistic service that addressed these needs.

This holistic approach has been particularly emphasised by Aboriginal commentators and organisations.[82] It received its most telling endorsement in the *Bringing Them Home* report on the 'Stolen Generation', which detailed the health effects on Aboriginal people who suffered legislated family separation and institutionalisation.[83] A solely clinical practice not only fails to recognise Indigenous perceptions of wellbeing, but also fails to address the origins of the desperate health needs of many Aboriginal people.

Disparate perceptions of healthworker practice have created conflict and confusion for both healthworkers and the health professionals with whom they work. This study points to the necessity for healthworker practice to be defined clearly, as either clinical extension or as client-centred holistic casework.

A way forward

At the policy level, a broad or holistic view of healthworker practice has endured for over twenty-five years. In general terms, this approach is both curative and preventive. Even though broader interpretations of healthworker practice have failed to transpire at the service delivery level, healthworkers have consistently advocated a need for wider engagement.

There are convincing arguments for formulating a holistic practice able to accommodate effectively the complexity and diversity of health risks faced by Aboriginal people. Client demand requires that healthworker practice address multiple health problems, including basic clinical ailments, the progression of chronic diseases, inadequate housing, transportation, income and food shortages, potential disruptions to medication schedules and the stresses of family life. Although previous policies have advocated that healthworkers also mobilise community action or development, equal grounds exist for a strategic casework approach focused on clients and their families.

A casework approach, based on home visits, synonymous with the client-centred holistic practice of Family Care healthworkers, provides services that are highly accessible to clients. By accommodating the negotiated health priorities of both the Indigenous client and the Indigenous healthworker, both the focus of the service and its mode of delivery retain a high degree of acceptability and cultural appropriateness. In particular, this approach accommodates crucial cultural health determinants described in the *Bringing Them Home* report, such as mistrust, fear, lack of responsiveness, dependency, exploitation and abuse.[84] It also aims to empower clients to take control of their own health. The client-centred approach based on home visits establishes a close relationship between the healthworker and the client, and familiarises the healthworker with the client's world. Positioned alongside the client, the healthworker is potentially able to activate the client's support network through supporting the client's efforts or advocating on their behalf.

Not only is a client-centred holistic practice manifestly accessible, acceptable and culturally appropriate, but it also embodies other first principles of primary health care, such as a focus on individuals and families, practicality, self-determination, participation, inter-sectorial collaboration and capacity building.[85] It engages dignity, self-esteem and self-reliance, social justice and a whole-of-life approach to health, as advocated in the landmark National Aboriginal Health Strategy.[86] For Aboriginal Health Services similar to the one in this study, it accords with the aspiration (quoted in the mission statement of the AHS in this study) to increase the life expectancy and health of the Aboriginal community through the development of *appropriate Aboriginal health care*.

While the National Aboriginal Health Strategy advocated a 'whole-of-life' view of health,[87] and numerous subsequent reports have advocated a holistic '*approach*',[88] the articulation of a complementary holistic Aboriginal healthworker *practice* has been missing. Aboriginal health-workers within this study have attempted to fill this gap through their documentation of a client-centred holistic practice.

Reorienting support, supervision and training

This study shows that the implementation of a client-centred holistic practice requires substantial organisational and professional support. Family Care healthworkers themselves proposed a set of practice guide-lines (covering eligibility for services, scope of services, hours of service, the responsibilities of both service provider and client and a detailed, negotiated care plan) as a basis to negotiate service provision with their clients. However, other health professionals and managers failed to fully understand either the complexities of their practice or their need for substantial support. The *Bringing Them Home* report also recom-mended comprehensive professional support and supervision for health-workers dealing with issues of social and emotional wellbeing.[89]

The need for support and guidance from a practitioner who has had experience working in a similar way with Indigenous clients is another finding of this study. While some nurses have sufficiently expanded their practice framework beyond a clinical focus to offer the necessary support, those lacking community-based primary health care experience and training are unlikely to benefit holistic healthworkers. The complex cultural components of the work—such as maintaining a non-dependent, enabling relationship with the client—have an emotional component that requires skilful debriefing. Appropriate supervision is mandatory for focused, systematic client-centred work.

Ongoing training and professional development are essential supports for healthworkers engaging a holistic practice. Currently, healthworkers appear less than adequately trained to skilfully handle the complexity of this work. The capacity to engage trust and at the same time avoid fostering client dependency demands well-developed negotiating and bargaining skills. The distinction between situations requiring either advocacy on behalf of the client or support for the client to advocate on their own behalf demands fine judgement and basic coaching skills. Recognition of shifts in client capacity due to familial and social disruption requires keen observation and consistent monitoring practices. The *Bringing Them Home* report highlighted the massive inter-generational effects of family disruption.[90] Healthworkers need ongoing development of their family work skills.

The client-centred holistic practice described within this study also has significant implications for healthworker training institutions. This approach requires a shift away from in-depth, curative clinical knowledge towards more sophisticated professional competencies relating to strategies of prevention. Because of the complexities and continuously shifting emphases in the work, initial training is not sufficient, and a systematic ongoing professional development programme is necessary.

The present study also indicates that a holistic healthworker practice requires substantial organisational and professional recognition in order to provide healthworkers with the requisite level of status to effectively complete their work. It also requires the complementary orientation of other health professionals who must, in particular, understand how healthworker practice intersects with their own activities—in order to avoid diverting the focus of healthworkers. Clear orientation to a holistic practice, and realistic expectations by professional colleagues, are likely to vastly improve healthworker morale and reduce resignations.

A comprehensive primary health care approach

Although the comprehensive primary health care strategy and broad approach advocated by the National Strategic Framework for Aboriginal and Torres Strait Islander Health is official policy of the federal Office of Aboriginal and Torres Strait Islander Health, this office still directs significant funding towards selective vertical programmes focused on specific diseases and conditions. Often these programmes employ healthworkers who focus narrowly on the particular health condition targeted by the programme; practice then remains largely clinical extension, albeit more specific. Nevertheless, the recent national reports on Indigenous health suggests that socio-economic status, social and cultural factors, access to good quality health care, environmental factors and specific lifestyle choices are the major influences on Aboriginal health.[91] Rather than healthworkers being confined to a narrow clinical focus in specific vertical programmes, a broader holistic practice engages them with these larger determinants of health status.

Holistic healthworker practice needs to be clearly defined within a co-ordinated, systematic, comprehensive primary health care approach to Aboriginal health. The numerous health professionals engaged in Aboriginal health programmes require a clear understanding of the approach, of Aboriginal healthworkers' potential contributions, and of where healthworkers are positioned in relation to them and their clients.

A client-centred holistic practice with a casework focus positions healthworkers alongside clients. From this standpoint, healthworkers are able to provide a continuum of care and to activate a client's support network. The familiarity and rapport of a healthworker, and their larger view of both client need and available supports, places them in the ideal position to co-ordinate care, both with doctors, nurses and social workers and with the family.

Where healthworkers encounter family relationships that are abusive of clients, they have the potential to initiate change by means of appropriate professional and organisational support and their community networks. Networks developed through a holistic practice also provide appropriately trained healthworkers with the potential to facilitate community action on shared prevention issues. Such a role positions Aboriginal healthworkers as professionals able to co-ordinate interventions directed at specific family and community concerns, which are often the genesis of wider health issues.

While there have been continuous efforts to 'professionalise' Aboriginal healthworker practice in the past decade, through the development of career pathways, portability of training, registration boards and healthworker associations, they have often been top-down efforts that fail to locate healthworker practice within a broader primary health care approach. Acknowledgement, systematic support and further development of a client-centred holistic healthworker practice would establish this practice as the basis for professional recognition. It is crucial that professional identity is founded on a distinct practice that is widely recognised to be applicable to a particular situation. The practice of Family Care healthworkers models a singular professional approach to the complex array of factors impairing the health of Aboriginal people. Rather than auxiliary status, it requires recognition as a vital component of a systematic approach to an effective health service. A shift to a recognised client-centred holistic practice has significant institutional and organisational implications.

Shifting organisational culture

If we heed the suggestions of the healthworkers in this study and re-fashion healthworker practice, there will be major implications for all institutions and organisations involved in Aboriginal health. At the policy level, revision will most likely require refocusing programmes and, within them, the healthworker role. Programme planners, in particular those planning vertical, disease-specific interventions, may have to change their plans for healthworkers. At the service delivery level, organisations may have to rethink their deployment of health-workers.

A shift in healthworker practice has significant implications for the strategic direction and corporate planning of Aboriginal primary health services. At the service level, a change in organisational focus is required. While curative clinical care is now the major focus of most Aboriginal health services, the promotion of a client-centred holistic healthworker practice would require equal attention to holistic preventive casework. Whereas a clinical focus gives clinical health professionals significant authority and influence in the development of policy, programmes and practices, a client-centred, holistic focus will require leadership from appropriately experienced Aboriginal healthworkers. This would enhance healthworker status relative to other health professionals. Such a change represents a significant transformation in organisational culture.

A professionally guided, systematic process of participatory organisational change would be necessary to facilitate such a cultural transformation. Within Aboriginal health agencies, such a process of organisational change would require the participation of managers, nurses, doctors, healthworkers and other employees. Ideally this process would establish an organisational understanding of healthworker practice and the rationale for its use as a primary vehicle of service delivery. Within this study, the healthworkers attempted to initiate such a process themselves, but lacked the necessary organisational support. Their unsuccessful attempt signals the need for a co-ordinated commitment to change processes.

An appropriate change process would enable participants to understand the multi-dimensional nature of a client-centred holistic practice, its collaborative style, and its requirement for integration with other services and ongoing staff training. Skilfully implemented, such a process would overcome organisational perceptions of healthworkers as clinical assistants or lackeys and endorse their legitimacy as unique professional practitioners.

Integration into the mainstream health and welfare arena would also be necessary. The healthworkers in this study undertook a multi-sectorial approach. Hence, they engaged with a variety of external health and welfare support workers, particularly those who interacted with Aboriginal families. These external workers require an awareness of both the orientation of the organisation delivering the health services and of holistic healthworker practice. Organisational development processes need to include outside personnel linked to healthworkers and their clients.

Managed organisational change, such as raising the awareness of a client-centred holistic healthworker practice, requires a serious financial commitment. This study has shown the need for enhanced professional development, mentoring and supervision opportunities. These have major implications for recruitment strategies and budgets.

In summary, history shows the need for a broader approach to complement the existing clinical programmes within Aboriginal Health Services. Doctors and nurses focus on clinical matters because their training provides them with the necessary expertise. A broader focus on prevention and the social and emotional wellbeing of clients is necessary to change Aboriginal health status. With appropriate organisational and professional support, Aboriginal healthworkers can make a major contribution. Ideally, the operations of Aboriginal health services should integrate curative clinical management and holistic prevention.

Acknowledgement and systematic support for a holistic prevention practice delivered by healthworkers would provide recognition and legitimacy for a distinct Indigenous professional health practice. Such recognition would embrace the unique understanding of healthworkers and use it to expand the knowledge base of Indigenous health practice.

Valuing healthworker knowledge

This study reveals how Aboriginal healthworkers extend the scope of Indigenous health practice to engage social, cultural and psychological health determinants particular to the Indigenous context. The collective body of knowledge of healthworkers includes specific health factors, how they manifest in the lives of clients, and strategies for intervention. Healthworker knowledge is a resource important to the professional status of healthworkers and to the professional development of everyone engaged with Indigenous health.

The *Bringing Them Home* report provided a detailed analysis of the history of the forced removal of Aboriginal children from their families and of the inter-generational effects on health.[92] It showed that within the Aboriginal community, almost every family bears the social, cultural and psychological scars of this legislation. The report made a significant contribution towards understanding the broader factors affecting Indigenous health status and the complex situations encountered by Aboriginal healthworkers. Likewise, I have provided detailed accounts of healthworkers engaged with these complexities. Their experience offers a wealth of knowledge concerning day-to-day factors affecting the health of Aboriginal people.

Extensive epidemiological data on Aboriginal health records the prevalence and incidence of disease and illness according to a range of demographic variables, but far less is known about the underlying social and cultural determinants of health that operate in the day-to-day context of people's lives. Healthworkers working beyond the clinic become familiar with this everyday experience. They witness first-hand the impact of a mix of detrimental social, cultural and psychological factors. Healthworkers have an extensive, collective repository of knowledge that is of vital importance to efforts to improve Aboriginal health.

It is important for other health professionals to recognise not only the practice of healthworkers, but also the knowledge and understandings generated within their practice. Professional recognition of healthworker knowledge would include valuing their contribution to policy and programme planning. The participation of healthworkers in planning would add an important dimension to understanding the effects of programmes at the community level. As long as healthworkers are denied professional recognition, status and participation in these forums, their knowledge remains under-utilised.

By incorporating healthworkers' knowledge into health education and training programmes, deeper understandings of the broader factors affecting Indigenous health can be shared with a wider audience. Other professionals require extensive orientation in order to work in Aboriginal health, and the experience and knowledge of healthworkers would add another dimension to their professional development programmes and provides a basis for establishing collegiate relationships.

While medicine has moved fast in the area of technical innovations, much work needs to be done on improving health services for Aboriginal people. Technical sophistication is considerable, but making services more accessible, acceptable and appropriate is still problematic. Aboriginal healthworkers are in a position to make a significant contribution to this area. Through trial and error, many have developed innovative practices of potential benefit to other health professionals.

Aboriginal organisations and government reports have consistently cited the need for the cultural orientation of health professionals working within the arena of Aboriginal health.[93] By building an archive of healthworker knowledge, health professionals can receive not only a cultural orientation, but also a deep understanding of the complex interaction of social, cultural and psychological health determinants affecting Aboriginal health.

Formal recognition of the particular understandings and practices developed by healthworkers—their body of professional knowledge—is an essential step towards legitimising them as unique professional practitioners. Training courses for healthworkers are well established all over the country, and building this formal body of knowledge promises increased training resources and enhanced training curricula. Such a process will also strengthen healthworker practice, their profession and its status amongst other health professionals.

Conclusion

Aboriginal health status continues to decline in comparison to the non-Aboriginal population in Australia. This poor status cannot be addressed effectively without acknowledging and incorporating the knowledge and understandings of healthworkers operating 'beyond the clinic'. For a long time, programmes and resources have focused on medical services and clinical management, and attempts to meet the social, cultural and environmental needs of Aboriginal people have been relatively under-resourced. There is a crucial need to balance clinical interventions with more holistic programmes.

The time, energy and skills devoted by committed doctors and nurses to clinical management projects in Aboriginal health desperately need to be complemented with more effective prevention strategies. Systematic approaches to prevention, drawing on family, community and professional networks, are necessary. The client-centred holistic practice of Aboriginal healthworkers, with full organisational and professional support, may provide the means. However, it will only be possible if healthworkers receive due recognition by inclusion in the planning and development of policies, programmes and practices.

The implications of this study, specific to site as it is, are clearly relevant to healthworkers around Australia. I suspect that they may also be relevant to many primary health workers elsewhere. The inadequate health status of Aboriginal people is magnified in less developed countries and diasporas around the world. Equally, local people in these contexts have knowledge and understandings vital to their own struggle. Perhaps I can finish as I began, and leave the last word with Ruby, who reminds us of an Indigenous healthworker's struggle:

> They wanted all us healthworkers 'cause we were going to change everything, but we're so strictly dictated to, it's changed nothing. Some of us have great ideas, and we could do it all, but we just can't do it. Instead of like handing things to us, we're always dictated to … People are still dying—Teddy's going to get his toes cut off, Daisy died … people are just dying of things that could have been changed.

Notes

Foreword

1 National Aboriginal and Torres Strait Islander Health Council, *National Strategic Framework for Aboriginal and Torres Strait Islander Health*, 2003.
2 Australian Health Ministers Advisory Council, Standing Committee on Aboriginal and Torres Strait Islander Health, *Aboriginal and Torres Strait Islander Health Workforce National Strategic Framework*, 2002.

Preface

1 Australian Bureau of Statistics and Australian Institute for Health and Welfare, *The Health and Wellbeing of Australia's Aboriginal and Torres Strait Islander Peoples*, p. 6.
2 ibid., pp. 137, 192; Australian Medical Association, *Public Report Card 2003: Aboriginal and Torres Strait Islander Health—Time for Action*, p. 12.
3 Kamien, 'Cultural Chasm and Chaos in the Health Care Services to Aborigines in Rural NSW'; Couzos and Murray, *Aboriginal Primary Health Care*, p. 5; Anderson, 'Towards a Koori Healing Practice'.
4 Rigney, *Internationalisation of an Indigenous, Anti-Colonial Cultural Critique of Research Methodologies*; Smith, *Decolonising Methodologies*; VicHealth Koori Health Research and Community Development Unit, *We don't like research … but in Koori hands it could make a difference*.

Chapter 1: At the Frontline

1 Royal Commission into Aboriginal Deaths in Custody, *National Report*, vol. 4; Australian Health Ministers Advisory Council, *Health Is life*; Human Rights and Equal Opportunity Commission, *Bringing Them Home*.
2 Royal Commission into Aboriginal Deaths in Custody, *National Report*, vol. 4, p. 228.

3 Australian Health Ministers Advisory Council, *Health Is life*.

4 Walt, *Community Health Workers in National Programmes*, p. 19.

5 Sidel and Sidel, 'Health Care Delivery System of the People's Republic of China'.

6 UNICEF and World Health Organization, *Final Report on the International Conference on Primary Health Care* (Alma Ata Declaration).

7 Walt, *Community Health Workers in National Programmes*, pp. 10–14.

8 World Health Organization, *The Primary Health Worker*, p. 4.

9 Walt, *Community Health Workers in National Programmes*, p. 21; Berman, 'Village Health Workers in Java, Indonesia'.

10 Soong et al., 'A Formula for Aboriginal Health Workers'; Willis, 'Has the Primary Health Worker Program Been Successfully Exported to the Northern Territory?'; Mayman, 'Why Joan Winch Needs $680,000'.

11 Saggers and Gray, *The Health of Aboriginal Australia*, p. 161.

12 Soong et al., 'A Formula for Aboriginal Health Workers', p. 21.

13 ibid.; Soong, 'Developing the Role of Primary Health Workers (Aboriginal) in the Northern Territory'; Hargrave, 'Focus on Aboriginal Health'; Devanesen, 'The Aboriginal Health Worker Training Program in Central Australia'; Soong, 'Aboriginal Health Workers in Australia'; Soong, 'The Role of Aboriginal Health Workers as Cultural Brokers'; Fleming and Devanesen, *Health Policies and the Development of Aboriginal Self-Management in the Northern Territory*, p. 4.

14 Soong, 'Developing the Role of Primary Health Workers (Aboriginal) in the Northern Territory', p. 29.

15 World Health Organization, *The Primary Health Worker*, p. 5.

16 Myers, *Pintupi Country, Pintupi Self*, pp. 277–9; Folds, 'Constraints on the Role of Aboriginal Health and Education Workers as Community Developers'.

17 Willis, 'Has the Primary Health Worker Been Successfully Exported to the Northern Territory?'; Willis, 'From Stonequist to Foucault?'.

18 Soong, 'The Role of Aboriginal Health Workers as Cultural Brokers', p. 270.

19 Winch, quoted in Ellis, 'Linking Our Future', pp. 8–16; Armstrong et al., *Review of Health Worker Education in Western Australia*, p. 11; Saggers and Gray, *The Health of Aboriginal Australia*, p. 161.

20 Ellis, 'Linking Our Future', p. 10.

21 Frankel, 'Peripheral Health Workers Are Central to PHC'.

22 ibid., p. 286.

23 Davidson, 'Training Amerindian PHC Workers'.

24 Cumper and Vaughan, 'Community Health Aides at the Cross-roads'.

25 Nichter, 'The Primary Health Care Centre as a Social System'.

26 Skeet, 'Community Health Workers', p. 294.

27   Berman et al., 1987, 'Community Based Health Workers', p. 457; Walt,
      'CHWs'; Walt, *Community Health Workers in National Programmes*, p. 45.
28   Walt, *Community Health Workers in National Programmes?*, pp. 26–8.
29   Walt, 'CHWs', p. 15.
30   Willis, 'From Stonequist to Foucault?', p. 65.
31   Bell, 'Health Maintenance in a Central Australian Community'; Myers,
      Pintupi Country, Pintupi Self, p. 277; Folds, 'Constraints on the Role of
      Aboriginal Health and Education Workers as Community Developers', p. 230.
32   Nathan and Japanangka, *Health Business*, p. 149.
33   Tynan, 'Women in the Health Role'.
34   Folds, 'Constraints on the Role of Aboriginal Health and Education Workers
      as Community Developers', p. 229.
35   Dixon et al., *A Career Structure for Aboriginal Health Workers in the Northern
      Territory*.
36   Armstrong et al., *Review of Health Worker Education in Western Australia*,
      pp. 1–63.
37   Soong, 'Developing the Role of Primary Health Workers (Aboriginal) in the
      Northern Territory', pp. 29–31.
38   Anderson, *Koorie Health in Koorie Hands*, p. 115; National Aboriginal
      Health Strategy Working Party, *A National Aboriginal Health Strategy*,
      pp. 85–6.
39   National Aboriginal Health Strategy Working Party, *A National Aboriginal
      Health Strategy*, p. x.
40   Ellis, 'Aboriginal and Islander Healthworkers Spread the Word', p. 12, my
      emphasis.
41   See Aboriginal Health Unit, *Aboriginal Health Worker Needs Analysis
      Reports—Kununurra, Broome, Carnarvon, Meekatharra, Blackstone (Central
      Desert), Kalgoorlie, Perth/Wheatbelt, Katanning*; Health Department of
      Western Australia, *Competencies for Aboriginal Healthworkers*; National
      Community Services and Health Industry Training and Advisory Board,
      *Aboriginal Health Worker and Torres Strait Islander Health Worker National
      Competency Standards Levels A to D*, draft.
42   Skeet, 'Community Health Workers', p. 294.
43   Franks and Curr, *Why Don't They Stay?*, p. 10.
44   ibid., p. 12; Josif and Elderton, *Working Together?* p. 30; Kirkby, *Roles and
      Relationships of Health Care Staff in Remote Kimberley Aboriginal
      Communities*, p. 15.
45   Aboriginal Health Ministers' Advisory Council, *Aboriginal and Torres Strait
      Islander Health Workers, Nurses and Doctors*, p. 12.
46   See Health Department of Western Australia, *Competencies for Aboriginal
      Healthworkers;* Gray, *Associate Diploma of Aboriginal Health*; Aboriginal
      Health Unit, *Associate Diploma in Aboriginal Health: Course Overview*.

47 Tsey and Scrimgeour, 'The Funder-Purchaser-Provider Model and Aboriginal Health Care Provision'.

48 Forrest, 'The Case For and Against the Concept of Specialist versus Generalist Health Workers'.

49 Tregenza and Abbott, *Rhetoric and Reality*, p. 8.

50 Dixon et al. *A Career Structure for Aboriginal Health Workers in the Northern Territory*, p. 25; Franks and Curr, *Why Don't They Stay?*, p. 11; Josif and Elderton, *Working Together?*, pp. 20–56; Kirkby, *Roles and Relationships of Health Care Staff in Remote Kimberley Aboriginal Communities*, pp. 18–41; Tregenza and Abbott, *Rhetoric and Reality*, pp. 7, 8.

51 Hart, 'Problems Facing Aboriginal Health Workers in a Community Health Service'; Cresap Pty Ltd, *Review of Health and Community Services*, p. 125; Franks and Curr, *Why Don't They Stay?*, p. 19; Josif and Elderton, *Working Together?*, p. 46; Kirkby, *Roles and Relationships of Health Care Staff in Remote Kimberley Aboriginal Communities*, p. 28; Tregenza and Abbott, *Rhetoric and Reality*, p. 62.

52 See Gray, *Associate Diploma of Aboriginal Health*; S. Bushby, personal communication, November 2001.

Chapter 2: Grassroots Healthworker Practice

1 Haebich, *For Their Own Good*.

2 M. Campbell, personal communication, May 1996.

Chapter 5: Genesis of a Healing Practice?

1 Hart, 'Problems Facing Aboriginal Health Workers in a Community Health Service', p. 16; Dixon et al., *A Career Structure for Aboriginal Health Workers in the Northern Territory*, p. 12; Franks and Curr, *Why Don't They Stay?*, p. 11; Josif and Elderton, *Working Together?*, p. 34; Kirkby, *Roles and Relationships of Health Care Staff in Remote Kimberley Aboriginal Communities*, pp. i–viii; Tregenza and Abbott, *Rhetoric and Reality*, p. 6.

2 Soong, 'The Role of Aboriginal Health Workers as Cultural Brokers', p. 270.

3 Tregenza and Abbott, *Rhetoric and Reality*, p. 22; Willis, 'From Stonequist to Foucault?', p. 69.

4 Anderson, *Koorie Health in Koorie Hands*, pp. 109–14; Anderson, 'Towards a Koori Healing Practice', pp. 39–42.

5 Anderson, *Koori Health in Koori Hands*; National Aboriginal Health Strategy Working Party, *A National Aboriginal Health Strategy*.

6 Dixon et al., *A Career Structure for Aboriginal Health Workers in the Northern*

Territory, p. 19; Josif and Elderton, *Working Together?*, p. 22; Kirkby, *Roles and Relationships of Health Care Staff in Remote Kimberley Aboriginal Communities*, p. 26; Abbott and Fry, *The Role of the Aboriginal Health Worker*, p. 3.

7   Ellis, 'Aboriginal and Islander Healthworkers Spread the Word', p. 12; Josif and Elderton, *Working Together?*, p. 22; Tregenza and Abbott, *Rhetoric and Reality*, p. 13.

8   Royal Commission into Aboriginal Deaths in Custody, *National Report*; Australian Health Ministers Advisory Council, Standing Committee on Family and Community Affairs, *Health Is Life*; Australian Bureau of Statistics and Australian Institute for Health and Welfare, *The Health and Wellbeing of Australia's Aboriginal and Torres Strait Islander Peoples*.

9   Josif and Elderton, *Working Together?*, p. 22; Franks and Curr, *Why Don't They Stay?*, p. 10.

10   Flick, 'Aboriginal Health Workers'; McMasters, 'Research from an Aboriginal Health Worker's Point of View'; Tregenza and Abbott, *Rhetoric and Reality*, p. 7.

11   Flick, 'Aboriginal Health Workers', p. 10.

12   Dixon et al., *A Career Structure for Aboriginal Health Workers in the Northern Territory*, p. 12; Ellis, 'Aboriginal and Islander Healthworkers Spread the Word', p. 12; Josif and Elderton, *Working Together?*, p. 22; Tregenza and Abbott, *Rhetoric and Reality*, p. 7.

13   Kirkby, *Roles and Relationships of Health Care Staff in Remote Kimberley Aboriginal Communities*, p. 26; Tregenza and Abbott, *Rhetoric and Reality*, p. 26.

14   Hunter, 'Stains on the Caring Mantle'; National Inquiry into the Separation of Aboriginal and Torres Strait Islander Children from Their Families, <www.austlii.edu.au/au/special/rsjproject/rsjlibrary/hreoc/stolen/stolen20.html>, accessed 27 June 2005.

15   Josif and Elderton, *Working Together?*, p. 21.

16   Ellis, 'Report of the Second National Aboriginal and Torres Strait Islander Health Worker Conference', p. 46.

17   Folds, 'Constraints on the Role of Aboriginal Health and Education Workers as Community Developers', p. 230.

18   Bell, 'Health Maintenance in a Central Australian Community', p. 205; Myers, *Pintupi Country, Pintupi Self*, p. 277; Nathan and Japanangka, *Health Business*, p. 149; Tynan, 'Women in the Health Role', p. 93; Franks and Curr, *Why Don't They Stay?*, p. 11; Soong, 'The Role of Aboriginal Health Workers as Cultural Brokers', p. 269.

19   Dixon et al., *A Career Structure for Aboriginal Health Workers in the Northern Territory*, p. 12.

20 McMasters, 'Research from an Aboriginal Health Worker's Point of View', p. 319.

21 Myers, *Pintupi Country, Pintupi Self*, p. 278; Tynan, 'Women in the Health Role', p. 93; Hunter, 'Aboriginal Mental Health Awareness'.

22 Tregenza and Abbott, *Rhetoric and Reality*, p. 37.

23 Dixon et al., A Career Structure for Aboriginal Health Workers in the Northern Territory, p. 12; Josif and Elderton, *Working Together?*, p. 49; Windsor, 'Workplace Bullying'.

24 Hart, 'Problems Facing Aboriginal Health Workers in a Community Health Service', p. 16; Franks and Curr, *Why Don't They Stay?*, p. 11; Josif and Elderton, *Working Together?*, p. 49.

25 Tregenza and Abbott, *Rhetoric and Reality*, p. 7.

26 Tsey, 'Aboriginal Health Workers'.

27 Soong et al., 'A Formula for Aboriginal Health Workers'.

28 Hargrave, 'Focus on Aboriginal Health', p. 575.

29 Devanesen, 'The Aboriginal Health Worker Training Program in Central Australia', p. 15; Fleming and Devanesen, *Health Policies and the Development of Aboriginal Self-Management in the Northern Territory*, p. 2.

30 Anderson, *Koorie Health in Koorie Hands*, p. 114.

31 National Aboriginal Health Strategy Working Party, *A National Aboriginal Health Strategy*, p. 85.

32 Aboriginal Health Ministers' Advisory Council, *Aboriginal and Torres Strait Islander Health Workers, Nurses and Doctors*, p. 9; National Aboriginal Health Strategy Evaluation Committee, *The National Aboriginal Health Strategy*, p. 75.

33 Office for Aboriginal and Torres Strait Islander Health Services, 'Progress Report on Responses to the Recommendations of the 1997 National Aboriginal and Torres Strait Islander Health Worker's Conference', p. 15.

34 Woolridge, 'A National Project to Benefit Health Workers', p. 3.

35 Fleming and Devanesen, *Health Policies and the Development of Aboriginal Self-Management in the Northern Territory*, p. 10; Kirkby, *Roles and Relation ships of Health Care Staff in Remote Kimberley Aboriginal Communities*, p. 41; Cordell, *The Career Structure of Aboriginal Health Workers within the Health Department of Western Australia*, p. 31.

36 Willis, 'From Stonequist to Foucault?', p. 65.

37 Soong, 'Developing the Role of Primary Health Workers (Aboriginal) in the Northern Territory', p. 30.

38 Hart, 'Problems Facing Aboriginal Health Workers in a Community Health Service', p. 16.

39 Armstrong et al., *Review of Health Worker Education in Western Australia*, p. 7.
40 Soong, 'Aboriginal Health Workers in Australia', p. 168; Dixon et al., *A Career Structure for Aboriginal Health Workers in the Northern Territory*, p. 25; Willis, 'From Stonequist to Foucault?', p. 65.
41 Soong, 'The Role of Aboriginal Health Workers as Cultural Brokers', p. 272; Atkinson, *Aboriginal and Torres Strait Islander Health Worker Training in WA*, p. 4.
42 Hart, 'Problems Facing Aboriginal Health Workers in a Community Health Service', p. 16.
43 Kirkby, *Roles and Relationships of Health Care Staff in Remote Kimberley Aboriginal Communities*, p. 23.
44 Walt, *Community Health Workers in National Programmes*, p. 53; Josif and Elderton, *Working Together?*, p. 30; Kirkby, *Roles and Relationships of Health Care Staff in Remote Kimberley Aboriginal Communities*, p. 17; Tregenza and Abbott, *Rhetoric and Reality*, p. 26.
45 Jackson et al., 'Towards (Re)conciliation'.
46 Tregenza and Abbott, *Rhetoric and Reality*, p. 15; Windsor, 'Workplace Bullying', p. 6.
47 Tregenza and Abbott, *Rhetoric and Reality*, p. 28.
48 Bradley, *Nursing Insights*, p. 26.
49 Nathan and Japanangka, *Health Business*, p. 149.
50 Armstrong et al., *Review of Health Worker Education in Western Australia*, p. 8; Dixon et al., *A Career Structure for Aboriginal Health Workers in the Northern Territory*, p. 7; Aboriginal Health Ministers' Advisory Council, *Aboriginal and Torres Strait Islander Health Workers, Nurses and Doctors*, p. 47; Josif and Elderton, *Working Together?*, p. 35; Hecker, 'Participatory Action Research as a Strategy for Empowering Aboriginal Health Workers'; Abbott and Fry, *The Role of the Aboriginal Health Worker*, p. 4; Tsey, 'Aboriginal Health Workers: Agents of Change?', p. 228.
51 Josif and Elderton, *Working Together?*, p. 8.
52 Franks and Curr, *Why Don't They Stay?*, p. 12; Dollard et al., 'Aboriginal Health Worker Status in South Australia'.
53 Flick, 'Aboriginal Health Workers', p. 10.
54 Tregenza and Abbott, *Rhetoric and Reality*, p. 23.
55 Hecker, 'Participatory Action Research as a Strategy for Empowering Aboriginal Health Workers', p. 784.
56 Scrimgeour, *Community Control of Aboriginal Health Services in the Northern Territory*, p. 93.
57 Hart, 'Problems Facing Aboriginal Health Workers in a Community Health Service', p. 16; Cordell, *The Career Structure of Aboriginal Health*

Workers within the Health Department of Western Australia, p. 10; Dolley, *Aboriginal Healthworker Career Structure*.

58 Kirkby, *Roles and Relationships of Health Care Staff in Remote Kimberley Aboriginal Communities*, p. 40.

59 Fleming and Devanesen, *Health Policies and the Development of Aboriginal Self-Management in the Northern Territory*, p. 4.

60 Cresap Pty Ltd, *Review of Health and Community Services*, p. 125.

61 See Dixon et al., *A Career Structure for Aboriginal Health Workers in the Northern Territory*.

62 Franks and Curr, *Why Don't They Stay?*; Josif and Elderton, *Working Together?*

63 Tregenza and Abbott, *Rhetoric and Reality*, p. 4.

64 Hart, 'Problems Facing Aboriginal Health Workers in a Community Health Service', p. 16.

65 Tregenza and Abbott, *Rhetoric and Reality*, p. 13; Hecker, 'Participatory Action Research as a Strategy for Empowering Aboriginal Health Workers', p. 787.

66 Tregenza and Abbott, *Rhetoric and Reality*, p. 14; Dixon et al., *A Career Structure for Aboriginal Health Workers in the Northern Territory*, p. 12.

67 Josif and Elderton, *Working Together?*, pp. 56–9; Kirkby, *Roles and Relationships of Health Care Staff in Remote Kimberley Aboriginal Communities*, p. 41.

68 Tregenza and Abbott, *Rhetoric and Reality*, p. 15; Josif and Elderton, *Working Together?*, p. 30; Franks and Curr, *Why Don't They Stay?*, p. 12; Hecker, 'Participatory Action Research as a Strategy for Empowering Aboriginal Health Workers', p. 786.

69 Kirkby, *Roles and Relationships of Health Care Staff in Remote Kimberley Aboriginal Communities*, p. 17.

70 Dixon et al., *A Career Structure for Aboriginal Health Workers in the Northern Territory*, p. 12; Franks and Curr, *Why Don't They Stay?*, p. 11.

71 Hart, 'Problems Facing Aboriginal Health Workers in a Community Health Service', p. 16; Dixon et al., *A Career Structure for Aboriginal Health Workers in the Northern Territory*, p. 25; Josif and Elderton, *Working Together?*, p. 46; Franks and Curr, *Why Don't They Stay?*, p. 11; Tregenza and Abbott, *Rhetoric and Reality*, pp. 7–8.

72 Josif and Elderton, *Working Together?*, p. 49.

73 National Aboriginal Health Strategy Working Party, *A National Aboriginal Health Strategy*, p. 85.

74 UNICEF and World Health Organization, *Final Report on the International Conference on Primary Health Care*, p. 5.

75 ibid., p. 15.

76 National Aboriginal Health Strategy Working Party, *A National Aboriginal*

Health Strategy, p. x; National Aboriginal and Torres Strait Islander Health Council, *National Strategic Framework for Aboriginal and Torres Strait Islander Health*, p. 2.

77 World Health Organization, *The Primary Health Worker*, p. 3.

78 Soong, 'Developing the Role of Primary Health Workers (Aboriginal) in the Northern Territory', p. 29.

79 Walsh and Warren, 'Selective Primary Care'; Rifkin and Walt, 'Why Health Improves'.

80 Berman et al., 'Community Based Health Workers', p. 457; Skeet, 'Community Health Workers', p. 294; Walt, *Community Health Workers in National Programmes*, p. 45.

81 Aboriginal Health Ministers' Advisory Council, *Aboriginal and Torres Strait Islander Health Workers, Nurses and Doctors*, pp. 9–12; Josif and Elderton, *Working Together?*, pp. 21–6; Franks and Curr, *Why Don't They Stay?*, p. 7; Tregenza and Abbott, *Rhetoric and Reality*, pp. 6–8.

82 Anderson, 'Towards a Koori Healing Practice', p. 41; Anderson, 'The National Aboriginal Health Strategy'; Tregenza and Abbott, *Rhetoric and Reality*, p. 14; Swan and Raphael, *Ways Forward*, p. 9.

83 Human Rights and Equal Opportunity Commission, *Bringing Them Home*: <www.austlii.edu.au/au/special/rsjproject/rsjlibrary/hreoc/stolen/stolen27.html>, accessed 27 June 2005.

84 ibid.

85 UNICEF and World Health Organization, *Final Report on the International Conference on Primary Health Care*, pp. 5–15.

86 National Aboriginal Health Strategy Working Party, *The National Aboriginal Health Strategy*, p. ix.

87 ibid., p. x.

88 Swan and Raphael, *Ways Forward*, p. 9; Human Rights and Equal Opportunity Commission, *Bringing Them Home*, p. 387; National Aboriginal and Torres Strait Islander Health Council, *National Aboriginal and Torres Strait Islander Health Strategy*, p. xiv; National Aboriginal and Torres Strait Islander Health Council, *National Strategic Framework for Aboriginal and Torres Strait Islander Health*, p. 2.

89 National Inquiry into the Separation of Aboriginal and Torres Strait Islander Children from Their Families, <www.austlii.edu.au/au/special/rsjproject/rsjlibrary/hreoc/stolen/stolen27.html>, accessed 27 June 2005.

90 ibid.

91 Australian Health Ministers Advisory Council, Standing Committee on Family and Community Affairs, *Health Is Life*; Australian Bureau of Statistics and Australian / Institute for Health and Welfare, *The Health and Wellbeing of Australia's Aboriginal and Torres Strait Islander Peoples*, pp. 133–45.

92   Human Rights and Equal Opportunity Commission, *Bringing Them Home*, p. 8.

93   Royal Commission into Aboriginal Deaths in Custody, *National Report*, p. 232; National Inquiry into the Separation of Aboriginal and Torres Strait Islander Children from Their Families, <www.austlii.edu.au/au/special/rsjproject/rsjlibrary/hreoc/stolen/stolen27.html>, accessed 27 June 2005; Australian Health Ministers Advisory Council, Standing Committee on Family and Community Affairs, *Health is Life*, p. 8; Australian Health Ministers Advisory Council, Standing Committee on Aboriginal and Torres Strait Islander Health, *Aboriginal and Torres Strait Islander Health Workforce National Strategic Framework*, p. 11.

Bibliography

Abbott, K. and D. Fry, *The Role of the Aboriginal Health Worker: AHWs Need Community Based Training and Traineeships*, Central Australian and Barkly Aboriginal Health Worker Association, Alice Springs, 1998.

Aboriginal Health Unit, *Aboriginal Health Needs Analysis Reports: Kununurra, Broome, Carnarvon, Meekatharra, Blackstone (Central Desert), Kalgoorlie, Perth/Wheatbelt, Katanning, WA*, Centre for Aboriginal Studies, Curtin University, Perth, 1991.

——*Associate Diploma in Aboriginal Health: Course Overview*, Curtin University, Perth, 1992.

Anderson, I., *Koorie Health in Koorie Hands*, Koorie Health Unit, Health Department of Victoria, Melbourne 1988.

——'Towards a Koori Healing Practice', in *Voices from the Land: The 1993 Boyer Lectures*, ABC Books, Sydney, 1993, pp. 30–44.

——'The National Aboriginal Health Strategy', in H. Gardner (ed.), *Health Policy in Australia*, Oxford University Press, Melbourne, 1997, pp. 119–35.

Armstrong, C., D. Gray, I. Wronski, B. Williams and D. Collard, *Review of Health Worker Education in Western Australia*, Department of Aboriginal Affairs, Perth, 1987.

Atkinson, D., *Aboriginal and Torres Strait Islander Health Worker Training in WA*, Centre for Aboriginal Medical and Dental Health, University of Western Australia, Perth, 2000.

Australian Bureau of Statistics and Australian / Institute for Health and Welfare, *The Health and Wellbeing of Australia's Aboriginal and Torres Strait Islander Peoples*, Australian Bureau of Statistics, Canberra, 2005.

Australian Health Ministers Advisory Council, *Aboriginal and Torres Strait Islander Health Workers, Nurses and Doctors: Roles and Relationships in Remote Australia*, Australian Health Ministers Advisory Council, Canberra, 1994.

——Standing Committee on *Aboriginal and Torres Strait Islander Health, Aboriginal Torres Strait Islander Health Workforce National Strategic Framework*, National Aboriginal and Torres Strait Islander Health Council, Canberra, 2002.

——Standing Committee on Family and Community Affairs, *Health Is Life: Report on the Inquiry into Indigenous Health*, Australian Health Ministers Advisory Council, Canberra, 2002.

Australian Medical Association, *Public Report Card 2003: Aboriginal and Torres Strait Islander Health—Time for Action*, Australian Medical Association, Canberra, 2003.

Bell, D., 'Health Maintenance in a Central Australian Community', in J. Reid (ed.), *Body, Land and Spirit*, University of Queensland Press, Brisbane, 1982, pp. 197–224.

Berman, P., 'Village Health Workers in Java, Indonesia: Coverage and Equity', *Social Science and Medicine*, vol. 19, no. 4, 1984, pp. 279–90.

Berman, P. A., G. R. Davidson and S. E. Burger, 'Community Based Health Workers: Head Start or False Start for All?', *Social Science and Medicine*, vol. 25, no. 5, 1987, pp. 443–9.

Bhaba, H. K., 'Cultural Diversity and Cultural Differences', in B. Ashcroft, G. Griffiths and H. Tiffin (eds), *The Post-Colonial Studies Reader*, Routledge, London, 1995, pp. 206–9.

Bradley, H., *Nursing Insights: Remote Area Health Care—Inside Perspectives of an Outsider*, Faculty of Nursing, University of South Australia, Adelaide, 1998.

Clifford, J., 'On Ethnographic Allegory', in J. Clifford and G. E. Marcus (eds), *Writing Culture: The Poetics and Politics of Ethnography*, University of California Press, Berkeley, 1986, 98–121.

Cordell, D., *The Career Structure of Aboriginal Health Workers within the*

Health Department of Western Australia: A Policy Analysis and Critique, MA thesis, University of Western Australia, 1995.

Couzos, S. and R. Murray, *Aboriginal Primary Health Care*, Oxford University Press, Melbourne, 1999.

Cresap Pty Ltd, *Review of Health and Community Services*, Department of Health and Community Services, Darwin, 1991.

Cumper, G. C. and J. P. Vaughan, 'Community Health Aides at the Cross-roads', *World Health Forum*, vol. 6, 1985, pp. 365–7.

Davidson, J. R., 'Training Amerindian PHC Workers: Evaluation of Government Training of Aguaruna (Jivaro) Traditional Birth Attendants', *Medical Anthropology*, vol. 9, no. 1, 1985, pp. 65–83.

Denzin, N. K., *Interpretive Interactionism*, Sage, Newbury Park, 1989.

——*Interpretive Ethnography*, Sage, Thousand Oaks, 1997.

Devanesen, D., 'The Aboriginal Health Worker Training Program in Central Australia', *Panacea*, vol. 13, no. 1, 1982, pp. 14–22.

Dixon, B., A. Kelly and B. Kirke, *A Career Structure for Aboriginal Health Workers in the Northern Territory*, Northern Territory Health, Darwin, 1987.

Dollard, J., T. Stewart, J. Fuller and I. Blue, 'Aboriginal Health Worker Status in South Australia', *Aboriginal and Islander Health Worker Journal*, vol. 25, no. 1, 1987, pp. 28–30.

Dolley, P., *Aboriginal Healthworker Career Structure: Review of Implementation*, Health Department of Western Australia, Perth, 1996.

Ellis, R., 'Aboriginal and Islander Healthworkers Spread the Word', *Aboriginal and Islander Healthworker*, vol. 14, no. 1, 1990, pp. 12–13.

——'Report of the Second National Aboriginal and Torres Strait Islander Health Worker Conference: "Uniting Our Voices"', *Aboriginal and Islander Health Worker Journal*, vol. 21, no. 3, 1997, pp. 10–18.

——'"Linking Our Future": The Third National Aboriginal and Torres Strait Islander Health Worker's Conference', *Aboriginal and Islander Health Worker Journal*, vol. 23, 1999, pp. 8–16.

Fine, M., 'Working the Hyphens: Reinventing Self and Other in Qualitative Research', in N. K. Denzin and Y. S. Lincoln (eds),

The Handbook of Qualitative Research, Sage, Thousand Oaks, 1994, pp. 70–82.

Fleming, K. and D. Devanesen, *Health Policies and the Development of Aboriginal Self-Management in the Northern Territory*, Northern Territory Department of Health, Darwin, 1985.

Flick, B., 'Aboriginal Health Workers: Slaves or Miracle Workers?', *Aboriginal and Islander Health Worker Journal*, vol. 19, no. 3, 1995, pp. 10–11.

Folds, R., 'Constraints on the Role of Aboriginal Health and Education Workers as Community Developers', *Australian Journal of Social Issues*, vol. 20, no. 3, 1985, pp. 228–33.

Forrest, B., 'The Case For and Against the Concept of Specialist versus Generalist Health Workers', *Aboriginal and Islander Health Worker Journal*, vol. 19, no. 4, 1995, pp. 28–30.

Frankel, S., 'Peripheral Health Workers are Central to PHC: Lessons from Papua New Guinea's Aid Posts', *Social Science and Medicine*, vol. 19, no. 4, 1984, pp. 279–90.

Franks, C. and B. Curr, *Why Don't They Stay?*, Northern Territory Department of Health and Community Services, Darwin, 1992.

Gray, E., *Associate Diploma of Aboriginal Health*, Marr Mooditj Aboriginal Health College, Perth, 1994.

Haebich, A. *For Their Own Good*, University of Western Australia Press, Perth, 1988.

Hall, S., 'The Work of Representation', in S. Hall (ed.), *Representation: Cultural Representations and Signifying Practices*, Sage, London, 1997, pp. 17–42.

Haraway, D. J., *Simians, Cyborgs and Women: The Reinvention of Nature*, Routledge, New York, 1991.

Hargrave, J., 'Focus on Aboriginal Health', *Medical Journal of Australia*, no. 2, 1981, pp. 575–6.

Hart, G., 'Problems Facing Aboriginal Health Workers in a Community Health Service', *Medical Journal of Australia, special supplement*, no. 1, 1981, pp. 15–16.

Health Department of Western Australia, *Competencies for Aboriginal Healthworkers*, Health Department of Western Australia, Perth, c.1993.

Hecker, R., 'Participatory Action Research as a Strategy for Empowering Aboriginal Health Workers', *Australian and New Zealand Journal of Public Health*, vol. 21, no. 7, 1997, pp. 784–8.

Human Rights and Equal Opportunity Commission, *Bringing Them Home: Report of the National Inquiry into the Separation of Aboriginal and Torres Strait Islander Children from Their Families*, Human Rights and Equal Opportunity Commission, Canberra, 1997.

Hunter, E., 'Stains on the Caring Mantle: Doctors in Aboriginal Australia Have a History', *Australian Medical Journal*, no. 155, 1991, pp. 779–83.

——'Aboriginal Mental Health Awareness: An Overview—Levels of Responsibility for Aboriginal and Torres Strait Islander Healthworkers', *Aboriginal and Islander Healthworker Journal*, vol. 17, no. 2, 1993, pp. 16–19.

Jackson, D., W. Brady and I. Stein, 'Towards (Re)conciliation: (Re)constructing Relationships between Indigenous Health Workers and Nurses', *Journal of Advanced Nursing*, vol. 29, no. 1, 1999, pp. 97–103.

Josif, P. and K. Elderton, *Working Together? A Review of Aboriginal Health Workers: Recruitment and Retention in the Northern Territory's 'Top End'*, Department of Health and Community Services, Darwin, 1992.

Kamien, M., 'Cultural Chasm and Chaos in the Health Care Services to Aborigines in Rural NSW', *Medical Journal of Australia, special supplement*, no. 2, 1975, pp. 6–11.

Kelly, A. and S. Sewell, *With Head, Heart and Hand*, Boolarong, Brisbane, 1989.

Kirkby, E., *Roles and Relationships of Health Care Staff in Remote Kimberley Aboriginal Communities*, Health Department of Western Australia, Perth, 1994.

Lincoln, Y. and E. Guba, *Naturalistic Inquiry*, Sage, Newbury Park, 1985.

McLennan, W. and R. Madden, *The Health and Welfare of Australia's Aboriginal and Torres Strait Islander Peoples*, Australian Bureau of Statistics / Australian Institute for Health and Welfare, Canberra, 1999.

McMasters, A., 'Research from an Aboriginal Health Worker's Point of View', *Australian and New Zealand Journal of Public Health*, vol. 20, no. 3, 1996, pp. 319–20.

Marcus, G. E. and M. J. Fischer, *Anthropology as Social Critique: An Experimental Moment in the Human Sciences*, University of Chicago Press, Chigago, 1986.

Mayman, J., 'Why Joan Winch Needs $680,000', *Australian Society*, vol. 7, no. 1, 1988, pp. 22–3.

Mills, C. W., 'The Sociological Imagination', in C. Lemert (ed.), *Social Theory: The Multicultural and Classic Readings*, Westview, Boulder, 1993 [1959], pp. 379–82.

Myers, F. R., *Pintupi Country, Pintupi Self*, Australian Institute for Aboriginal Studies, Canberra, 1983.

Nathan, P. and D. L. Japanangka, *Health Business*, Heinemann, Melbourne, 1983.

National Aboriginal and Torres Strait Islander Health Council, *National Aboriginal and Torres Strait Islander Health Strategy*, Consultation Draft, National Aboriginal and Torres Strait Islander Health Council, Canberra, 2001

——*National Strategic Framework for Aboriginal and Torres Strait Islander Health: Framework for Action by Governments*, National Aboriginal and Torres Strait Islander Health Council, Canberra, 2003.

National Aboriginal Health Strategy Evaluation Committee, *The National Aboriginal Health Strategy: An Evaluation*, Department of Human Services and Health, Canberra, 1994.

National Aboriginal Health Strategy Working Party, *A National Aboriginal Health Strategy*, Australian Government Publishing Service, Canberra, 1989.

National Community Services and Health Industry Training and Advisory Board, *Aboriginal Health Worker and Torres Strait Islander Health Worker National Competency Standards Levels A to D*, draft, National Community Services and Health Industry Training and Advisory Board, Sydney, 1996.

National Health and Medical Research Council, *Guidelines on Ethical*

Matters in Aboriginal and Torres Strait Islander Health Research, National Health and Medical Research Council, Canberra, 1991.

——'Criteria of Health and Medical Research of Indigenous Australians', National Health and Medical Research Council, 2003, <www.nhmrc.gov.au/funding/advice.htm>, accessed 18 December 2003.

——*Values and Ethics: Guideline for Ethical Conduct in Aboriginal and Torres Strait Islander Health Research*, National Health and Medical Research Council, Canberra, 2003.

Nichter, M. A., 'The Primary Health Care Centre as a Social System: PHC, Social Status, and the Issue of Teamwork in South Asia', *Social Science and Medicine*, vol. 23, no. 4, 1986, pp. 347–55.

Office for Aboriginal and Torres Strait Islander Health Services, 'Progress Report on Responses to the Recommendations of the 1997 National Aboriginal and Torres Strait Islander Health Worker's Conference', *Aboriginal and Islander Health Worker Journal*, vol. 23, no. 3, 1999, pp. 14–22.

Patton, M. Q., *How to Use Qualitative Methods in Evaluation*, Sage, Beverley Hills, 1987.

Paul, B. D., *Health, Culture and Community*, Russell Sage, New York, 1955.

Rabinow, P., 'Representations are Social Facts', in J. Clifford and G. E. Marcus (eds), *Writing Culture: The Poetics and Politics of Ethnography*, University of California Press, Berkeley, 1986, pp. 234–61.

Rifkin, S. B. and G. Walt, 'Why Health Improves: Defining the Issues Concerning CPHC and SPHC', *Social Science and Medicine*, vol. 23, no. 6, 1986, pp. 559–66.

Rigney, L. R., *Internationalisation of an Indigenous, Anti-Colonial Cultural Critique of Research Methodologies: A Guide to Indigenist Research Methodology and its Principles*, HERDSA Annual International Conference, Adelaide, 1997.

Royal Commission into Aboriginal Deaths in Custody, *National Report*, vol. 4, Australian Government, Canberra, 1991.

Saggers, S. and D. Gray, *The Health of Aboriginal Australia*, Allen & Unwin, Sydney, 1991.

Said, E. W., 'Orientalism', in B. Ashcroft, G. Griffiths and H. Tiffin (eds), *The Post-Colonial Studies Reader*, Routledge, London, 1995, pp. 87–91.

Scrimgeour, D., *Community Control of Aboriginal Health Services in the Northern Territory*, Menzies School of Health Research, Darwin, 1997.

Sidel, J. and R. Sidel, 'Health Care Delivery System of the People's Republic of China', in K. Newell (ed), *Health by the People*, World Health Organisation, Geneva, 1975, pp. 1–12.

Skeet, M., 'Community Health Workers: Promoters or Inhibitors of Primary Health Care?', *World Health Forum*, vol. 5, no. 4, 1984, pp. 291–5.

Smith, D. E., *The Everyday World as Problematic*, Northeastern University Press, Boston, 1987.

Smith, L., *Decolonising Methodologies: Research and Indigenous People*, Zed Books, London, 1999.

Soong, F. S., 'Developing the Role of Primary Health Workers (Aboriginal) in the Northern Territory: A Challenge to the Health Professions', *New Doctor*, vol. 11, 1979, pp. 29–31.

——'Aboriginal Health Workers in Australia', *World Health Forum*, vol. 2, 1982, pp. 166–9.

——'The Role of Aboriginal Health Workers as Cultural Brokers: Some Findings and Their Implications', *Australian Journal of Social Issues*, vol. 18, no. 4, 1983, pp. 268–74.

Soong, F. S., B. Reid, M. Keller and L. Thompson, 'A Formula for Aboriginal Health Workers', *Australian Nursing Journal*, vol. 6, no. 4, 1976, pp. 21–3.

Spivak, G. C., 'Can the Subaltern Speak?', in B. Ashcroft, G. Griffiths and H. Tiffin (eds), *The Post-Colonial Studies Reader*, Routledge, London, 1995, pp. 24–8.

Spradley, J. P., *The Ethnographic Interview*, Holt, Rhinehart and Winston, London, 1979.

——*Participant Observation*, Holt, Rhinehart and Winston, New York, 1980.

Stringer, E., *Action Research: A Handbook for Practitioners*, Sage, Thousand Oaks, 1999.

Swan, P. and B. Raphael, *Ways Forward: National Aboriginal and Torres Strait Islander Mental Health Policy National Consultancy Report*, Australian Government Publishing Service, Canberra, 1995.

Tregenza, J. and K. Abbott, *Rhetoric and Reality: Perceptions of the Roles of Aboriginal Health Workers in Central Australia*, Central Australian Aboriginal Congress, Alice Springs, 1995.

Trinh, M. T., 'No Master Territories', in B. Ashcroft, G. Griffiths and H. Tiffin (eds), *The Post-Colonial Studies Reader*, Routledge, London, 1995, pp. 215–18.

Tsey, K., 'Aboriginal Health Workers: Agents of Change?', *Australian and New Zealand Journal of Public Health*, vol. 20, no. 3, 1996, pp. 227–9.

Tsey, K. and D. Scrimgeour, 'The Funder-Purchaser-Provider Model and Aboriginal Health Care Provision', *Australian and New Zealand Journal of Public Health*, vol. 20, no. 6, 1996, pp. 661–4.

Tyler, S. A., 'Post-Modern Ethnography', in J. Clifford and G. E. Marcus (eds), *Writing Culture: The Poetics and Politics of Ethnography*, University of California Press, Berkeley, 1986, pp. 122–40.

Tynan, B. J., 'Women in the Health Role', in F. Gale (ed.), *We Are Bosses Ourselves: The Status and Role of Aboriginal Women Today*, Institute for Aboriginal Studies, Canberra, 1983, pp. 93–9.

UNICEF and World Health Organization, *Final Report on the International Conference on Primary Health Care* (Alma Ata Declaration), World Health Organization, Geneva, 1978.

VicHealth Koori Health Research and Community Development Unit, *We don't like research … but in Koori hands it could make a difference*, VicHealth Koori Health Research and Community Development Unit, Melbourne, 2000.

Wadsworth, Y., *Everyday Evaluation on the Run*, Allen & Unwin, Sydney, 1997.

Walsh, J. A. and K. S. Warren, 'Selective Primary Care: An Interim Strategy for Disease Control in Developing Countries', *Social Science and Medicine*, vol. 14C, 1980, pp. 145–63.

Walt, G., 'CHWs: Are National Programmes in Crisis?', *Health Policy and Planning*, vol. 3, no. 1, 1988, pp. 1–21.

———*Community Health Workers in National Programmes: Just Another Pair of Hands?*, Open University Press, Bristol, 1990.

Willis, E., 'Has the Primary Health Worker Program Been Successfully Exported to the Northern Territory?', *Aboriginal Health Project Information Bulletin*, vol. 6, 1984, pp. 13–18.

———'From Stonequist to Foucault?: Theorising Interactions amongst Aboriginal Health Workers and Remote Area Nurses', in H. Keleher and F. McInerney (eds), *Nursing Matters: Critical Sociological Perspectives*, Harcourt Brace, Sydney, 1998, pp. 63–78.

Windsor, J., 'Workplace Bullying', *Aboriginal and Islander Health Worker Journal*, vol. 25, no. 3, 2001, pp. 4–9.

Woolridge, M., 'A National Project to Benefit Health Workers', *Aboriginal and Islander Health Worker Journal*, vol. 23, no. 2, 1999, pp. 2–3.

World Health Organization, *The Primary Health Worker: Working Guide, Guidelines for Training*, Pitman, London, 1980.

Index